Why Am I So Grumpy, Dopey And Sleepy?

What everyone must know about how to get more mental and physical energy.

by

Lorrie Medford, C.N.

LDN Publishing
P.O. Box 54007
Tulsa, Oklahoma 74155

WHY AM I SO GRUMPY, DOPEY AND SLEEPY?
What everyone must know about how to get more mental and physical energy.
ISBN #0-9676419-5-0

LDN Publishing
P. O. Box 54007
Tulsa, OK 74155

Second Printing

Library of Congress Cataloging-in-Publishing Data

Medford, Lorrie,

Why Am I So Grumpy, Dopey and Sleepy?
Lorrie Medford, C.N.
International Standard Book Number: 0-9676419-5-0
1. Nutrition 2. Health 3. Self Improvement I.Title

NOTE: This book is not intended to take the place of medical advice. Readers are advised to consult their doctor or other qualified healthcare professional regarding treatment of their medical conditions.

Printed in the United States of America

10 9 8 7 6 5 4 3 2

(For ordering information, refer to the back pages of this book.)

The names of my clients have been changed. Any similarity to a real person is purely coincidental.

Contents

Introduction: People Need Energy! 11

Part One: Do You Have An Energy Shortage?

1. Why Do People Get Chronically Fatigued? 17

Part Two: Why Am I So Grumpy?

2. How Does Stress Cause Adrenal Fatigue? 25

Part Three: Why Am I So Dopey?

3. Why Am I Depressed? 37
4. Why Am I Always Tired and Hungry? 47

Part Four: Why Am I So Sleepy?

5. Why Can't I Sleep? 57
6. Why Does Poor Digestion Cause Fatigue? 61

Part Five: Designing Your Life for Energy

7. What Should I Eat? 67
8. Ten Life Design Principles for Energy 77
9. What Vitamins Do I Need? 83
10. How Should I Live? 89
11. How Can I Get Started? 99

Endnotes 105

Index 109

Foreword

Lorrie has written an information-packed book for the person who complains of being tired and run down.

I first began to consult with Lorrie in April 2000 when I was experiencing occasional dizziness and a problem with low-blood sugar and sugar cravings. Within two weeks of my first appointment, the dizziness was gone, the cravings left, and my energy was better.

Lorrie has also helped me to have amazing energy while competing for Miss America, where I was 2nd runner-up. I've also learned that keeping my body well nourished and balanced helps me to stay healthy and perform better, even with all of the traveling required as Miss Oklahoma.

Lorrie's new book is written in a clear, easy-to-understand style and is based on her many years of experience as a nutritionist and researcher. As I read this book, I could see why Lorrie has been so successful in helping to restore health and energy to so many people. I highly recommend her book!

Casey Preslar
Miss Oklahoma 2002
Tulsa, Oklahoma

Acknowledgements

The people who helped me the most to put this book together are my precious clients, who so often tell me that their main reason for coming to see me is due to their fatigue. So, many thanks to my clients, especially those who have allowed me to share their stories in this book.

Also, special thanks go to Dr. Donna Smith, a practicing Certified Clinical Nutritionist, for her wonderful comments, suggestions and edit. I really appreciate all of the time you have taken out of your busy schedule to read my manuscript, Donna. You are talented both as a nutritionist and editor.

I'm grateful for health researches and authors Dr. Nancy Appleton and Dr. Bruce West. Thanks for your permission to quote you throughout this book. I'm also grateful to the other writers and health professionals, including Dr. John Lee, Dr. James Wilson, Dr. Diana Schwarzbein and the writings of nutritionist Dr. Royal Lee.

I'm always grateful to my own staff, Anne Spears and Carolyn Clark who manage to juggle client orders and appointments, while supporting the production of my books. Thank you both so much for all of your hard work and continual encouragement to write this book. Your gifts and friendship are so appreciated.

Many thanks to Lori Oller, for your edit. Your talent, focus and compassion are so appreciated.

I'm so aware that any of our gifts, talents and desires are all given to us from God. So finally, I thank God with all of my heart. Every morning as my staff and I pray, we are grateful to God to have jobs where we can impact people's lives with encouragement, knowledge and good nutrition.

About the Author

Author and motivational speaker, Lorrie Medford has a B.A. in Communications and is a licensed Certified Nutritionist from The American Health Science University (AHSU). She also holds certification as a personal trainer from The International Sports Science Association (ISSA). She is a member of the Oklahoma Speaker's Association and she also serves on the Advisory Board for Standard Process, Inc.

In addition to writing this book, she has also written *Why Can't I Stay Motivated?, Why Can't I Lose Weight?, Why Can't I Lose Weight Cookbook, Why Do I Need Whole-Food Supplements?, Why Do I Feel So Lousy?, Why Am I So Wacky?, Why Eat Like Jesus Ate?, and Why Do I Really Need Herbs?*

A health researcher and journalist, Lorrie has studied nutrition, whole-foods cooking, herbs, health, fitness, and motivation for more than 20 years. Lorrie taught her weight-loss class at a local junior college and through her own business for more than 10 years, and taught natural foods cooking classes in Spokane, Washington and Tulsa, Oklahoma for 5 years.

Lorrie has a rich history of community involvement teaching nutrition and is a sought-after speaker for civic groups, churches, hospitals, and wellness organizations. She shares her knowledge in her seminars, and through her thriving nutritional consultation practice, *Life Design Nutrition,* in Tulsa, Oklahoma.

She is uniquely qualified to write about health and fitness. Lorrie knows what it's like to be a *cranky calorie counter* obsessed with foods, dieting, and striving to be thin. After struggling with her weight for many years, Lorrie lost more than 35 pounds and has kept it off for more than eighteen years.

People Need Energy!

If you think you are the only one who complains of a personal energy crisis, take heart. Statistics show that nearly half of all Americans suffer from low energy. And the other half were apparently too tired to answer the survey!

Seriously, nine out of ten clients that I see tell me they lack energy. How bad is this lack of energy?

You know you're tired when you fill the car up with gas at the pump and try to pay with your library card! Or you go shopping with your spouse and you fall asleep in the parking lot. At home, you don't even have enough energy to find the remote control for your TV. Instead you stay on the warm couch and watch two hours of televised bowling or worse, infomercials. You know, the stuff that's "not available in stores." By the time they get to, "But wait, that's not all," you've already ordered $2,000 worth of stuff you don't even need!

And that's just physical tiredness. What about mental fatigue? Do you have brain fog by 3:00 p.m.? Or from 3:00 p.m. on, do you watch the clock until it's time to go home because you can't concentrate on work any more? Then when it's time to go home, you can't find your keys?

Are You Tired?

When I interview clients, I often ask them how they have been handling their lack of energy. A male client said, "I read and sleep a lot. I make myself get up to do things, but it's really hard." I like helping people enjoy their lives, and this usually means helping them have more energy!

Having enough energy is major! We need it to be productive, stay healthy, and to deal with life's circumstances. We can't enjoy life without energy. But unfortunately, most of us don't understand how our bodies work. As children, we are never taught about what could make us tired. As adults, we can either struggle with each day, or finally learn about how to get more energy. It's better later than never!

Lacking energy is universal. A common complaint I hear is: "There is so much that I want to do, but I'm always tired." Having energy can change your life. I know from personal experience. I've lost weight, but more importantly, I've gained my energy back. I've also helped thousands of people with their energy crises. Here are some of their comments:

Connie said, "I now can stay awake after dinner! Before I came to see you, I used to barely have enough energy to make dinner, and I would fall asleep on the couch. The supplements and eating plan have helped me tremendously."

Mary Jane reported, "I finally cleaned out the garage. My husband is amazed! I haven't had this much energy in years."

Kim said, "My depression is gone, and I finally have the energy to exercise. I've lost 25 pounds with Lorrie's help."

We're Supposed to Have Energy!

Did you realize that the normal state of health is to have energy? We were created to never have an energy shortage. Every part of our digestion and metabolism was designed to keep us active for a full, long life.

Drop in at your local day care and look at the children. They have so much energy, they are like the Energizer Bunny® they just keep going and going, and going. We should, too!

One of the most important functions of your body is to produce energy from the food you eat. When energy production declines, the result is fatigue. If you are tired, lethargic, run down, and/or fatigued, then your body is sending some clear messages that something is wrong! **Realize that low energy is a symptom of some health imbalance or syndrome.** In fact, fatigue is the first sign of biochemical imbalance due to vitamin deficiencies. If not corrected, it will lead to nutrition-related diseases.

Obviously, fatigue often occurs due to a poor diet or not getting enough sleep. Yet fatigue also accompanies many diseases from the common cold to heart disease or diabetes.

It's easy to assume that as we get older, we will just get more run down, because that's all we have ever heard about. "Oh, Shirley, just accept that you are tired. After all, you are not a teenager anymore." This is not true. I've helped many people regain their energy and they say that they feel better than they did as teenagers. (Thank goodness they didn't dye their hair pink or pierce any body parts!)

What Could Be Wrong?

When clients come to me with complaints of low energy, I become their energy detective. Below is a list of possible energy robbers. This list may be overwhelming, but as you'll see in this book, most are related to diet, nutrition and lifestyle.

Possible Causes of Fatigue

- Vitamin or mineral deficiencies
- Sluggish adrenals
- Hypoglycemia (low-blood sugar)
- Excess carbohydrates/sugars
- Allergies
- Anemia
- Poor digestion and malabsorption
- Celiac Sprue disease
- Poor diet
- Side effect of prescription drugs
- Heavy metal toxicity
- Mineral imbalance
- Chronic Fatigue Syndrome
- Sluggish thyroid
- Diabetes
- Sluggish liver
- Candida Albicans
- Excessive stress
- Constipation
- Epstein Barr virus
- Insomnia
- Toxic liver or bloodstream
- Hormone imbalance
- Negative thinking

You might be surprised to see negative thinking on this list. If you're one of those people who thinks the glass is half empty, you may be too tired to pick it up anyway!

Where Do You Need Help?

What about you? Do you jump out of bed with lots of energy? Do you feel like you are getting the most out of your life? Or do you come home from work exhausted? If so, let's find out why!

You **can** have more energy. You **can** wake up and not feel like you need to sleep four more hours. You don't have to be exhausted after work. Most people have energy leaks that are easily corrected.

Perhaps you just want to be more alert or more active. Or perhaps you suffer from depression, pain or insomnia. So often people treat these symptoms with anti-depressants, pain medications or sleep medications, thinking that there is no other choice. But I've discovered in working with so many clients that we can do much better than just live with or mask these symptoms. We can find the causes by looking at nutritional components, and then making lifestyle changes to reverse the problem.

No matter who you are, or what the cause is for your lack of energy, the ideas and suggestions in this book will help you to get healthy. **Getting your energy back is more than just a health issue; it's a life issue!**

From my work with thousands of clients, I've found that most people's fatigue is related to: adrenal, thyroid, or low-blood sugar issues. You'll understand why using stimulants such as caffeine and sugar set us up for further fatigue. And you'll learn how vital it is to know if you have any nutritional deficiencies which cause fatigue.

Here is a list of the parts of this book and their chapters.

Part One gives you a general overview of the many, many reasons why people get fatigued and how to know if you may suffer from Chronic Fatigue (CFS) or Fibromyalgia (FMS) Syndromes. You may not be that tired, or, you may know someone who has Chronic Fatigue or Fibromyalgia. Either way, you'll see that there are many causes and more importantly, many solutions.

Part Two gives an overview of the adrenal glands, how vital they are for health, and how our fast-paced, stressful lifestyle sets us up for adrenal fatigue. You'll also learn how high-insulin levels contribute to stress, disease, weight gain and fatigue.

Part Three looks at fatigue related to the thyroid gland and depression. It also tells you how improving your blood-sugar levels increases your energy.

Part Four looks at the nature and cause of sleep problems and the effect of medications on sleep. We'll also look at the relationship between digestion, antibiotics and fatigue.

Part Five gives you practical tips for creating more energy in your life. You'll learn the Ten Life Design Principles, how to eat for optimal energy and how to understand vitamins and their link to energy leaks. We'll also give you tips for stress management, better sleep and regular exercise.

Finally, I wrap up the book with a short chapter on how to get started with basic steps to get you going, a recap of recommended nutritional supplements and meal planning tips.

Throughout this book, I'll refer you to "natural" health professionals. These include: Naturopathic Doctors (N.D.), Certified Nutritionists (C.N.), Certified Clinical Nutritionists (C.C.N.), and doctors (D.C., M.D., D.D., D.O., D.D.S., Ph.D.) who have studied Clinical Nutrition.

I've also included Endnotes and an Index for those who would like to do additional research. Let's get started on your journey to energy and vitality.

PART ONE

Do You Have an Energy Shortage?

Chapter One

Why Do People Get Chronically Fatigued?

In my office, we have so many requests for help with fatigue, that we have an "Energy Hotline." Here's how it goes.

• If your idea of a happy hour is not a cocktail, but a 15-minute nap, press one.

• If you go on vacation and your energy runs out before your money, press two.

• If listening to this message has worn you out, press three and go back to bed!

Perhaps you're tired. Even too tired to read this book! Never mind. You can be helped! I used to be a depressed, cranky, calorie counter who never exercised and had to drag myself out of bed every day. I've changed and you can, too.

Did you know that over 25 million Americans have severe fatigue (lasting at least one month) at any given time?[1]

Fatigue has been such a common complaint, that every client who comes to my office fills out several pages of paperwork to help discover nutritional links to fatigue. I also use various nutritional biochemical testing including saliva testing or blood tests to discover any vitamin and mineral deficiencies. Throughout the years I've also found nutritional tests and questionnaires such as a health and symptom history extremely valuable for identifying hidden health problems. They often give us clues to causes for fatigue.

Why Are You Tired?

Most of us have days when we lack some sleep because of a barking dog, crying child or snoring spouse. After a few days we feel better. But what about the people who **never** feel better? Day after day they drag on. They complain of brain fog. Listlessness. Lack of concentration. How did they get that way? And more importantly, what can they do?

You might just have occasional fatigue. But Americans are so tired that in 1988, there actually became a name for a real disease which has been acknowledged as becoming a national epidemic. The Centers for Disease Control (CDC) defined a syndrome they called Chronic Fatigue Syndrome (CFS) which refers to fatigue that doesn't go away with normal bed rest.

Formerly, CFS was known as Chronic Epstein Barr Virus Syndrome. Since there is no one "medical" examination for CFS, to meet their definition, most physicians diagnose CFS based upon this criteria: a patient must have debilitating fatigue for six months or more and have at least eight of these "unexplained" symptoms.[2]

- Severe fatigue for at least 6 months
- Low-grade fever or chills
- Unexplained muscle weakness
- Fatigue that lingers after exercise
- Loss of concentration/depression
- Sleep disturbances
- Recurrent sore throats
- Swollen lymph nodes
- Joint pain
- Headaches
- Muscle pain
- Sudden onset of symptoms

Taking this quick test below may help you know if your fatigue could be related to CFS.

Nutrition Test #1

1. Do you get infections like the flu, colds, and sore throats easily?
2. Do you have depression and/or anxiety?
3. Do you experience muscle pain and joint pain?
4. Do you have recurring headaches?
5. Do you have any sleep disorders?
6. Do you often have a low-grade fever?

7. Do you have swollen lymph nodes?
8. Do you experience lack of concentration?
9. Do you have problems with your digestion or colon?
10. Do you have severe fatigue?

If you answered the majority of these statements with yes, you may have CFS. More than 50 million people have been diagnosed with Chronic Fatigue Syndrome. No wonder coffee houses are springing up on every corner in the U.S.!

How Do We Get CFS?

For some time, people have called CFS a mystery, with no one clear cause—it just happens all of a sudden. I've found that the causes are varied and many. Here are some possible causes I've discovered from my research.

Dr. Ronald L. Hoffman, author of *Tired All the Time*, believes CFS is probably due to viruses, yeasts, allergies, chemical and heavy metal poisons, stress and hormone imbalances.[3]

Dr. Jacob Teitelbaum in his book, *From Fatigued to Fantastic,* believes that people with CFS have a combination of several problems but some common patterns are infections, disrupted sleep and hormonal imbalances.[4]

According to authors of *The Immune System Cure*, Lorna Vanderhaeghe and Dr. Patrick Bouic, parasites play a major role in the development of CFS weakening the body which has serious long-term health implications.[5]

What I've also found is that people who come to see me who have already been diagnosed with CFS have such problems as: ongoing stress and adrenal fatigue, poor digestion, diabetes, heart disease, malabsorption, hypothyroidism, hypoglycemia, anemia, food allergies, yeast issues, or multiple nutritional deficiencies. Poor diet and exposure to pollutants in the air and water are linked as well.

I've had to deal with different components, depending on each person, but nearly everyone I have seen with CFS has adrenal fatigue, thyroid fatigue and/or nutritional deficiencies. They weren't just tired; they were exhausted!

Because nothing shows up on traditional blood tests, several of my clients reported to me that their doctor said it must be something "in their head," and referred them on to a psychiatrist who would prescribe an anti-depressant. Just because it doesn't show on their tests doesn't mean it's not real. Traditional medical tests can't reveal nutritional deficiencies. So many fatigue problems include a nutritional component, and as you'll see throughout this book, it's an extremely important component.

CFS often becomes another type of condition involving fatigue accompanied with pain, called Fibromyalgia.

What About Fibromyalgia?

Fibromyalgia, according to Dr. Teitelbaum, currently affects nearly six million Americans.[6] Similar to CFS, Fibromyalgia is a syndrome characterized by tender knots called trigger points in the muscles. These knots cause aches, pain, sleep problems and unrelenting fatigue.

Diagnosis is based on a patient's complaints since a medical interpretation of blood tests and/or X-rays are frequently normal, thus they don't reveal anything.

In *The Fibromyalgia Handbook*, authors Harris McIlwain and Debra Bruce list common symptoms of Fibromyalgia as:[7]

- Pain
- Fatigue
- Morning stiffness
- Trigger points
- Sleep problems
- Anxiety
- Difficulty in concentration
- Depression
- Headaches
- Irritable bowel syndrome
- Urinary symptoms
- Painful menstrual cramps
- Discoloration of hands & feet
- Swelling, numbness and tingling in hands, arms, feet, and legs

According to the American College of Rheumatology, a person can be diagnosed with Fibromyalgia if they have: 1) Widespread aches and pain, and 2) Pain upon pressing at least 11 of the 18 trigger points on the body, also known as tender points.[8]

In his revised version of *Reversing Fibromyalgia,* Dr. Joe Elrod lists the vicious cycle of events and factors that contribute to both the onset and progression of Fibromyalgia.[9]

- Poor diet
- Nutritional deficiencies
- Accumulation of toxins
- Traumatic experiences
- Toxic cells
- Low growth hormone levels
- Lack of exercise
- Weakened immune system
- Infections
- Serotonin disruption
- Stress, anxiety and depression

I like Dr. Elrod's approach because it shows the relationship between our **lifestyle** and **disease.** While you may not have anything as serious as CFS or Fibromyalgia (FMS), you can see that not eating well or not getting enough sleep or exercise can set up the progression of even more severe health problems.

Some of my clients have done extremely well battling their Fibromyalgia. A client named Melissa who came to see me because of severe pain and fatigue says, "I was diagnosed with Fibromyalgia in 1998. After taking supplements that Lorrie suggested and eating better, every symptom was gone. If I eat right, like she told me, I have no symptoms. Yet the doctors told me that there was no help for it."

In an article entitled "Fibromyalgia and Synthetic Vitamins," researcher Dr. Bruce West says that if you have Fibromyalgia and you've taken handfuls of synthetic vitamins, you may be making yourself worse because high doses of synthetic vitamins can cause powerful nutritional deficiencies. He says that virtually all grocery store-bought vitamins are synthetic. Dr. West suggests that you eliminate all synthetic vitamins for 30 days and see for yourself whether or not there is a link to your pain.[10] (See my book *Why Do I Need Whole-Food Supplements?* listed at the back of this book for information on how to buy nutritional supplements.)

Hidden Food Allergies

In the same article, Dr. West lists other causes of Fibromyalgia as poor digestion, poor metabolism of sugar, and food allergies. Additionally, he says that if you have recurring hang nails, cracks in your heals or mouth along with Fibromyalgia, you have an essential fatty acid deficiency for which he recommends raw, organic flaxseed oil daily.[11]

Many of my clients could link food allergies to their fatigue and Fibromyalgia. I recommend Stephen Astor's book, *Hidden Food Allergies* which is an easy-to-read book to help you pinpoint your food allergies. Dr. Astor believes what you eat can make a difference and there are many documented cases where proper attention to food allergies alleviated a host of physical illnesses.[12]

Dr. Joseph Mercola is an Osteopathic Doctor who has an informative internet health site. Quoting from the Annual Meeting of the American College of Nutrition in Orlando, Florida, he reported a review of 17 Fibromyalgia patients who eliminated corn, wheat, dairy, citrus, soy and nuts. After two weeks without eating any of these potential food allergens, nearly half of the patients reported significant reduction of pain, and 76% of them reported a reduction in other symptoms, such as headache, fatigue, bloating, heartburn, and breathing difficulties.

After the food elimination phase of the study, the patients were then instructed to reintroduce one of these foods every two or three days and monitor their reaction to it.

Some of the reactions to foods were pain, headache, and gastrointestinal distress. The most common problem-causing foods or ingredients for the patients in this study were corn, wheat, dairy, and citrus.[13]

Is It Really Incurable?

Dr. Elrod reports that in the mainstream medical community, Fibromyalgia is considered incurable. (They rely on anti-depressants and anti-inflammatory drugs, but these offer only short-term relief.)[14] Since physicians can't point to a definite cause, it's hard for them to find a cure!

Yet, I've been delighted at the number of people who have come to me with symptoms of CFS or FMS who are better. Their energy has returned, their pain has subsided, and their depression has left. There are nutritional components to most fatigue and, therefore, many nutrition-related solutions.

What's the Bottom Line?

What do people with CFS and FMS have in common? Most have experienced some type of severe stress, whether it was physical stress, such as accidental injury, surgery or infection, or emotional stress, such as the loss of a loved one. Additionally, many were trying to get by on a diet of junk foods. Most have some type of allergy and/or digestive problems, constipation, or liver congestion which further cause fatigue. Often because of the poor diet and lack of sleep, they have low serotonin levels which further aggravate the condition. Now they are sleep deprived and depressed! And finally, most people with Fibromyalgia have multiple vitamin and mineral deficiencies.

Uh-oh! Where do you start? I recommend you see a "natural" health professional as listed on page 15 to be nutritionally tested so you know exactly what to take. Several supplements can make a great difference in increasing energy. For example, magnesium helps promote muscle relaxation and the entire B complex feeds the nervous system. Here are additional recommendations.

Recommended supplements:

·Antioxidants (vitamins A, C, E and selenium)

·Magnesium

·Vitamin B complex

·Folic acid/B12 and Iron (per test results)

·Essential oils

·Zinc and chromium

·Gymnema (Medi-Herb)

In Part Two, we'll see how stress affects your energy and your life, and its link to CFS and FMS.

PART TWO

Why Am I So Grumpy?

Chapter Two

How Does Stress Cause Adrenal Fatigue?

Stress is so pervasive that I wrote a quick test that I give in my office. How do you know you're stressed?

You know you're stressed when:

· You listen to your relaxation tapes on high speed.

· You take your shower with your panty hose still on.

· You start to brush your teeth, and the funny taste in your mouth makes you realize you are brushing your teeth with your husband's hair gel! That's stress!

Stress is everywhere. Tammy came to see me because she had constant migraines, a low sex drive and frequent colds. Vicki experienced major mood swings, and she could not lose weight. Andrea was tired, even when she had a good night's sleep, and she complained of brain fog. While their symptoms were different, their underlying problem was stress.

Your energy and even your attitude and productivity all depend on the health of your adrenal glands. **Nearly every chronically tired person has tired adrenal glands.** But more importantly, chronic stress is a significant factor which influences diseases such as Chronic Fatigue Syndrome and Fibromyalgia. Depression is also linked to stress.

Everyone is stressed, even teens. When I was a teenager, we all sat down and ate together as a family at night. Today families leave the house between 7 and 8 in the morning, often not returning until well past dinner. Eating out is their only option. Our fast-paced lifestyles cause us to eat fast food. A combination of not eating regular meals, and eating poorer quality food finally catches up with us. But that's not all. Stress can come from many directions and it all adds up.

Measured Stress

Dr. Thomas H. Holmes at the University of Washington School of Medicine developed a way to measure the amount of stress in an individual's life, called "The Holmes-Rabe Social Readjustment Rating Scale." Inspired by the work of Dr. Hans Seyle, it shows the relationship between stress and physical symptoms. For example, here are a few life situations and their numerical "points."

• Death of a spouse or other close family member	100
• Divorce	73
• Marital separation	65
• Jail term	63
• Personal injury or illness	53
• Marriage	50
• Fired from work	47
• Retirement	45

Imagine if you have several of these stressors simultaneously, as many people do. If you have less than 150 points, you only have a small chance of developing a stress-related illness. If you have between 151-300 points, you have a 50% chance of a major health breakdown in the next two years. If you have over 300 points, then it increases to an 80% chance of developing a major stress-related illness.[15] Stress matters!

You'll notice that even situations we consider happy such as marriage or retirement still rated high on stress.

What about you? Maybe you're not going through any of these, but we all have many other types of stressors.

Types of Stress

Emotional stressors include fear, depression, grief, hate and worry relating to relationships, finances and work issues.

Physical stressors include illness, chronic pain, sleep problems, overworking, surgery, or lack of exercise. Temperature extremes cause stress. Toxins—either environmental toxins, or toxins caused by invading microorganisms—all contribute to stress.

Dietary stressors include eating processed foods, caffeine, sugar and toxins, such as additives and preservatives. For example, eating a candy bar and a coke for breakfast, (Of course, you've never done that!) immediately stresses the adrenal glands for hours.

Interestingly, your adrenals respond to every kind of stress the same way, whatever the source. However, it's worse when many of these stressors occur simultaneously.

Our bodies were designed to handle the normal mild stresses of life. But if the stressors are extreme for long periods of time, like most people's constant, stressful lifestyle, that's when the affect of stress becomes chronic. Without adequate rest and nutrition to replenish the depleted vitamin and mineral stores, the adrenal stress just gets worse and the result is unrelenting fatigue.

These stressors don't necessarily have to be actual occurrences. Just worrying and thinking about a situation can cause an adrenal response, such as making a cold sales call, or asking someone out on a date. Just imagining a negative situation can even cause an adrenal response. Your nervous system can cause an emotional response that would be the same as a real situation. The greater the perceived stress, the greater the response.

For example, the other day I was looking for my car keys. All of a sudden, I thought that I locked them in my car. Immediately, my heart rate increased and blood rushed to my head. These were responses from my adrenal glands trying to help me deal with this stress. Luckily, my keys were in my pocket! But my body reacted as though they weren't.

So often my clients say, "I've been stressed like this for years. Why should I worry about it now?" We have far more stress today. Years ago this adrenal response meant the difference between life and death. Today adding stress such as drinking 20 cups of caffeine to our normal stressors can be as deadly.

The adrenals sit on top of your kidneys, and are as big as your thumb. They are incredibly important for releasing anti-stress hormones, but they are also involved with female hormone production and blood-sugar regulation. That's why women have hormone problems, such as irregular or stopped cycles when they are under stress. (Your body knows it's not wise to help an exhausted woman become pregnant!)

Our adrenal glands are the body's shock absorber that determines how we deal with stress. I've heard it likened to a car battery. If you kept your lights on all day, you might need a jump. But if the battery is too depleted, you need a new battery. For these people, a day of rest isn't enough. They may need three to six months to finally recover!

The stress response in the body is called the General Adaptation Syndrome. It has three stages: Alarm, Resistance and Exhaustion stages.

The Alarm stage is for a "fight or flight" response. You know, thousands of years ago when we needed a short burst of energy to run from a dinosaur or wild animal. This response speeds up the heart and makes you energetic. It's a quick, short-term response to stress. It was designed "for emergency only." If the reaction is successful, the body returns to normal. Unfortunately, today, due to all the types of stressors previously mentioned, we use the Alarm response over and over, and over, even unknowingly. Uh-oh!

The Danger of Stimulants

Today, all it takes to wear out this adrenal response is to indulge in a lifestyle of stimulants such as coffee, tea, sugar, soda, nicotine, alcohol or drugs. Combine that with overworking and lack of rest. We don't and can't even eat well enough to feed the adrenal glands to make up for long-term nutritional deficiencies and stress. Every time you push yourself beyond normal limits, you demand more of your weakened adrenal glands.

In the Resistance stage, the body adapts to the stress and slowly becomes more fatigued. It becomes harder to recover from a cold or flu. This can last months or even years.

This leads to the Exhaustion stage. In this stage, you're too tired to get out of bed. Your body lacks energy to contain the stress, so it breaks down. As nutrients are depleted, the heart muscle is weakened as well as the immune function. You may even experience depression, irritability, autoimmune disease, and/or heart disease. You also become vulnerable to every virus that comes around.

Stress and High-Cortisol Levels

The adrenal glands normally secrete hormones in a cycle, with the highest values in the morning and the lowest at night. Under prolonged stress, our adrenal glands secrete more of a hormone called cortisol, causing abnormally high levels which don't resume to normal cycle levels.

According to Dr. Diana Schwarzbein, author of *The Schwarzbein Principle II,* diseases linked with high-cortisol levels are: Type II diabetes, hypertension, stroke, osteoporosis, cholesterol abnormalities, depression and heart attacks.[16] Symptoms of high-cortisol levels include:

- Ankle swelling
- Anxiety and panic attacks
- Decreased energy
- Depression
- Fatigue
- Hair loss
- Headaches
- High-blood pressure
- High-cholesterol levels
- High blood-sugar levels
- Increased cravings for sugar
- Increased thirst
- Insomnia
- Impotence
- Irritability
- Loss of bone mass
- Lower back pain
- Weight gain around abdomen

Symptoms of Stress

We don't always recognize stress as it occurs. For that reason, we may not even be aware of how much stress we are under, especially, if we think that we can just handle it. We may think we are just handling it, but our adrenal glands are slowly and quietly becoming exhausted! Symptoms of severe stress are similar to symptoms of high-cortisol levels:

- Fatigue
- Anger
- Headaches
- Lowered resistance
- Low-blood sugar
- Insomnia
- Cravings
- Dizziness
- Depression
- Aches and pain
- Anxiety
- Low-blood pressure
- Weight gain

A stressful lifestyle can cause hypoglycemia, digestive problems, fatigue and low immune function, but almost anything can trigger the stress.

How stressed are you? Here's a quick test:

Nutrition Test #2

1. Do you crave salt?
2. Do you have depression?
3. Do you experience decreased ability to handle stress?
4. Do you have a low sex drive?
5. Do you have trouble getting up in the morning or trouble falling asleep at night?
6. Do you get dizzy when you stand up suddenly?
7. Do you take a long time to recover from illness?
8. Do you experience increased PMS?
9. Do you have problems with your memory and concentration?
10. Do you have unrelenting fatigue?
11. Do you have heartburn, indigestion or nausea?

If you answered yes to 8 or more, you may already have the beginning of some type of stress-induced illness. But it's not too late to turn it around!

Stress Causes Fatigue!

Stress is a major concern and cost. We spend 9.4 billion dollars a year to cope with stress. And the Centers for Disease Control reported that more than half of all deaths between the ages of one and 65 result from stressful lifestyles.

Because stress is an underlying factor in many diseases, medicines for stress are major selling drugs. Doctors first prescribed valium in 1963. Today, Americans spend $7 billion on anti-depressants per year.

There's no question that **stress causes fatigue**. So many disorders are linked to stress. According to Dr. James Wilson, author of *Adrenal Fatigue: The 21st Century Stress Syndrome,* adrenal fatigue is related to a long list of disorders: hypoglycemia, allergies, arthritic pain and decreased immune response, PMS, anxiety, depression, insomnia, respiratory infections, asthma, frequent colds, and full-blown diseases such as Fibromyalgia, Chronic Fatigue Syndrome, adult onset diabetes, alcoholism and auto-immune disorders.[17] Wow! Just reading that list could wear out your adrenal glands!

According to Maureen Salaman, author of *Your Health Questions Answered Naturally,* stress can even make you infertile. And up to 80% of health problems are stress related.[18]

Dr. Schwarzbein puts stress at the top of her list of things which raise insulin levels including: caffeine, alcohol, aspartame, tobacco, steroids, lack of exercise, and a low-protein diet, all which further cause fatigue.[19]

Why Hasn't My Doctor Helped?

Dr. Wilson explains that despite the fact that subclinical hypoadrenia (low-adrenal function) was recognized and treated earlier in the 20th century, it is almost invisible to modern medicine. Unfortunately, mainstream medicine doesn't recognize adrenal problems until it's too late and the adrenals are exhausted as in Addison's or Cushing's disease.[20] Yet nearly every client I've seen has some level of adrenal stress.

The only medical test to detect hypoadrenia are tests for Addison's disease. However, as a Clinical Nutritionist, there is a test that I've used successfully to indicate possible hypoadrenia. This is a saliva hormone test for two adrenal hormones: cortisol and DHEA (dehydroepiandrostenedione). Not only are these tests as valid as blood tests, but they have been written about in scientific journals and are even accepted by some insurance plans.

Dr. Wilson explains that in the last 50 years, pharmaceutical and insurance companies have altered the practice of medicine. Today, most doctors receive their income from insurance companies, and medical training is dependent on large drug companies for funding.[21] Prior to that time, a doctor used observations and physical examinations. He looked at your skin. He asked questions about your bowel movements and the color of your urine. He inquired about your sleep patterns and diet. He even asked you about your kid's soccer team. (No, I'm just kidding!) Doctors used to take more interest in your lifestyle as well.

Today drugs and/or surgery are the therapies offered by modern medicine. Patients are given an ICD (International Classification of Disease) code for their disease to classify their illness, or the insurance company doesn't pay. So if an illness doesn't show up on a lab test or fit a diagnostic code, or if there is no known drug treatment or reason to have surgery, then it's treated as though the problem is not real or does not exist. It's in your head. There is no ICD code for adrenal fatigue, so there is no approved medical therapy. Additionally, if the doctor doesn't use an approved medical therapy (drugs or surgery), there is no payment.[22]

So off you go to a "head doctor" or a psychiatrist who can write you a prescription for an anti-depressant. Yet no one in these fields looks at the nutritional or lifestyle causes and possible solutions.

Dr. Wilson also explains that until 1992, members of the American Medical Association (AMA) were forbidden to associate with practitioners of alternative medicine. Even today, information about therapeutic nutrition is still dismissed as being inferior to modern medicine.

However, I've found that it's impossible to solve a nutritional problem with a drug! Since medical doctors only receive one nutritional course in their years of education, how can they link disease to nutrition? Fortunately, more doctors are beginning to look into this question of alternative or complementary therapies, including nutritional therapy.

Here's a great example of how nutrition can help. My client, Lori, suffered from many classic symptoms of what the medical field categorizes as General Anxiety Disorder for several months before she came to see me with the problem. She experienced several symptoms, such as tingling in the feet, hands and lips, hair-loss, never-ending muscle tension, fatigue, dizzy spells, heart palpitations, skin sensitivity and general feelings of fear and anxiety. She remembers her struggle with the disease:

> I knew I had a serious problem because it was often keeping me from my daily activities, but I also knew that God did not want me to "cover up my symptoms" with drugs that my medical doctor might prescribe. Instead, He led me to Lorrie who immediately recognized the nutritional imbalances that were affecting my adrenals and thyroid. She recommended changes in my diet, such as eliminating sugar, coupled with lots of rest and moderate exercise. Whole-food supplementation, including the vitamin B complex for energy and minerals for relaxation, plus products to support my adrenals and thyroid, quickly put me on the right path to wholeness and healing. I find that I feel 100% better when I strictly follow the protocols Lorrie suggested.

Panic attacks, obsessive-compulsive disorders, eating disorders and phobias all have a nutritional component. While they require professional nutritional treatment, a healthy diet, adequate rest, moderate exercise, and stress management can help tremendously.

What Can You Do?

For proper adrenal health, you'll need to get adequate protein. Additionally, take adrenal-supportive supplements.

B vitamins are the single most important nutrient for the nervous system. The B vitamins affect immune functioning according to Dr. Leon Chaitow in his book, *You Don't Have To Die: Unraveling the AIDS Myth.*

He reports that Thiamine (B1) deficiency is linked to a decline in immune function, and a Riboflavin (B2) and Pyridoxine (B6) deficiency are required for antibody production. Pantothenic acid (B5) and Biotin help prevent viral infection, and B12 ensures T and B cell efficiency. Folic acid is vital for improving a weakened immune status.[23]

Theoretically, it is possible to acquire your B vitamins from a perfectly balanced diet. But in our society, where foods are grown in nutrient-deficient soil, plus stress and a poor diet make this almost impossible! The B vitamins help convert food to energy, and support mood control in the brain and nervous system. They are natural energy boosters.

According to Maureen Salaman, even moderate Thiamine B1 deficiency can cause anxiety or neuroses. Foods high in Thiamine are brewer's yeast, wheat germ, rice bran, whole grains, beans, peas and nuts. Green, leafy vegetables are high in the B complex vitamins and Folic acid. Pantothenic acid (B5) supports adrenal function. It's found in whole grains, cauliflower, broccoli, legumes and salmon.[24]

Caffeine, sugar, alcohol, and tobacco rob the body of B vitamins. So here is a list of things to eliminate: Stimulants such as coffee, chocolate, soda, refined white sugar, and food additives, such as MSG, nitrates, aspartame and alcohol. Most people go on fad diets to lose weight and get more energy, and then take these stimulants when they begin to experience fatigue. These stimulants cause fatigue!

A whole-food multiple vitamin and mineral is vital for everyone since American soils are dangerously deficient in minerals such as magnesium, chromium and manganese. Under stress, your body pulls minerals from your bones, teeth, hair and organs. That's why it's so important to eat well and take vitamin/minerals when under severe stress. Additionally, I recommend essential fatty acids.

A deficiency of magnesium can cause panic attacks, fatigue or insomnia. Good sources are green leafy vegetables, bananas, seafood, grains, nuts, and seeds. Magnesium also helps with muscle twitches and muscle tension.

Eleuthero Root, Panax Ginseng and Withania are safe herbs for improving the body's reaction to stress. Licorice Root is good if you don't have high blood pressure. (I use Medi-Herb which is only sold through health professionals.)

Antioxidants (vitamins A,C,E and selenium) are important when a body is under stress because it is more vulnerable to free radical damage. Antioxidants neutralize free radical damage. Vitamin C is extremely helpful for adequate production of the adrenal hormones.

Sources of vitamin C: apples, red peppers, oranges, broccoli, green peppers, and strawberries.

Sources of vitamin E: whole grains, almonds, beans, liver, leafy greens, and vegetable oils.

Sources of selenium: wheat germ and whole grains.

Sources of vitamin A: kale, sweet potato, carrot, squash, spinach, broccoli, pumpkin, and cantalope.

I carry professional supplements such as a desiccated adrenal product which is wonderful for adrenal support. You'll want to see your health care professional for them.

Recommended supplements:

·Vitamin B complex

·Magnesium

·Essential oils

·Eleuthero Root (Siberian Ginseng) (Medi-Herb)

·Panax Ginseng (Medi-Herb)

·Licorice Root (Medi-Herb)

·Withania (Ashwaganda by Medi-Herb)

·Antioxidants (vitamins A, C, E and selenium)

·Desiccated adrenal support

You'll also want to check your thyroid, which leads us to the next section about low thyroid function and fatigue.

PART THREE

Why Am I So Dopey?

Chapter Three

Why Am I Depressed?

Often people come to see me complaining of fatigue combined with what they call brain fog and/or depression. As if it were not enough that they are tired; now they can't remember what they were going into the kitchen to get, but they are so depressed, they don't care any more!

According to Dr. Wilson, 80% of people suffering from adrenal fatigue also have symptoms of low thyroid.[25] The adrenals and thyroid work together. If the adrenal glands are weak, the thyroid could slow down to compensate; this additionally causes low-blood pressure. I'll spend a lot of time on depression in this chapter, but let's start with a look at the relationship between the thyroid and fatigue.

Nearly 11 million Americans suffer from some degree of hypothyroidism. If you have three or more of the following symptoms, you may have a sluggish thyroid.

Nutrition Test #3

1. Do you have cold hands and feet?
2. Do you have trouble losing weight?
3. Do you have painful and irregular periods?
4. Do you have high cholesterol and triglycerides?
5. Do you have insomnia and fatigue?
6. Do you have trouble getting motivated to exercise?
7. Do you have uncommon hair loss or thinning hair?
8. Do you need caffeine and stimulants to make it through a day?
9. Do you have problems with depression and mental confusion?
10. Does your family have a history of low thyroid?
11. Do you have trouble with constipation?
12. Do you have dry, coarse skin or brittle nails?

Your body's metabolism depends on your thyroid. The thyroid produces the hormone thyroxine. If too much thyroxine is secreted, it causes high-thyroid function (hyperthyroidism). If not enough thyroxine is secreted, it causes low-thyroid function (hypothyroidism) which can lead to obesity. Here are symptoms of low-thyroid function:

- Fatigue
- Depression
- Mood swings
- Cold hands and feet
- Dry, lifeless hair
- Constipation, gas, bloat
- Menstrual irregularities
- Reduced initiative
- Brittle nails
- Weight gain
- Pale, dry skin
- Loss of eyebrow hair
- Thinning hair
- Ringing in the ears
- PMS, Heavy periods

Additionally, if uncorrected, hypothyroidism is linked to infertility and increased cholesterol levels.

How's Your Thyroid?

Over the past several years, people have come to my office because of a weight problem, stating that their blood tests for thyroid were perfect. In some cases, it was obvious that the person's thyroid function was impaired. But blood tests are often "normal" even if the thyroid gland is malfunctioning because these tests show how much thyroid hormone is circulating in the blood, not how much is in the cells. Up to 70% of thyroid function may be lost before blood tests become abnormal.[26]

In 1976, the late Dr. Broda O. Barnes, a world renowned thyroid expert, discussed the relationship between body temperature and the thyroid in her book, *Hypothyroidism: The Unsuspected Illness.* In her fascinating book, she links many problems to hypothyroidism including: migraines, emotional/behavior problems, infections, skin diseases, menstrual disorders, hypertension, heart attacks, arthritis, diabetes, hypoglycemia, obesity and aging.

She stated that as many as 40 percent of Americans had hypothyroidism. Even today, millions of people still have a "sluggish" thyroid.

Here is a simple and popular test developed by Dr. Barnes that you can use to determine if your thyroid is under-active.

The Barnes' Basal Temperature Test

1. Shake down thermometer and place it by your bed before retiring.
2. Upon awakening and before getting up, take your temperature under your arm and hold thermometer for 15 minutes being as still as possible.
3. Record the temperature and date.
4. Do this for 3 to 5 days in a row.

Your basal body temperature should be between 97.8° F. and 98.2° F. Anything lower can indicate hypothyroidism and anything higher could indicate hyperthyroidism.[27]

What Hurts Your Thyroid?

According to The Eck Institute newsletter which is based on the research of Paul Eck, there are many reasons for thyroid dysfunction including: copper or mercury toxicity, impaired cell permeability, toxicity from radiation, exhausted adrenals, flourides in drinking water which interfere with iodine metabolism, autonomic imbalances, oxidant stress or impaired fatty acid metabolism. Even foods, such as soy, and raw broccoli, cabbage and cauliflower may inhibit thyroid hormone utilization.[28]

Excess estrogen causes a hormonal imbalance that is linked to hypothyroidism. Eating foods that hinder the thyroid function makes you tired. Processed foods are toxic to the body. Here's a short list of the worst offenders:

- Coffee
- Sugar
- Cookies
- Cake
- Candy
- Soft drinks

We'll discuss nutritional solutions for the thyroid later in this chapter. Let's move on to depression.

Depression

Depression affects more than 17 million people every year just in the United States. Nutritionist Carol Simontacchi in her book, *Crazy Makers*, says that processed foods can physically erode our brains. She reports that the drug Prozac ranks fifth in the top ten pharmaceuticals, and over $7 billion is spent on anti-depressants per year. Sadly, the prescriptions for children, ages six to twelve, rose 209 percent in just one year.[29]

I've seen many causes for depression. For example, Mary came to me with complaints of fatigue and depression. She was diligent to make dietary changes and followed a "liver/colon cleanse." A month later her depression was completely eliminated.

A sluggish liver is related to depression. The two major detoxification pathways in the liver need foods such as Folic acid, the B complex, and antioxidants in Phase 1 and cruciferous vegetables such as broccoli, cabbage, Brussels sprouts, garlic, onions and kale in Phase 2. Without these wonderful healing foods, toxins find their way into the blood and into fatty parts of the body where they are stored for years. Many diseases including depression, high cholesterol and high-blood pressure are symptoms of a fatty, toxic liver. Many symptoms get treated while ignoring the underlying problem of a toxic liver. (See *Why Do I Feel So Lousy?*)

A client named Ilene wrote:

> I found Lorrie three years ago and began to follow her protocols. Since then she has helped my circulation, fibrous breast, and long-standing gum problems. However, I was still losing ground and I went to my medical doctor who diagnosed me with clinical depression. She recommended the drug, Effexor. Not wanting to take any drugs, I called Lorrie. She told me that historically St. John's Wort has been used for depression, but that she couldn't advise me to not take the drug, but to discuss it with my doctor. Before this I found it nearly

impossible to finish tasks. My sleep was interrupted. Following the St. John's Wort, my days began to come together. I finish tasks easily. And my purpose in life is clear again.

Another client, John, also came with a combination of fatigue and depression. After simply eliminating sugar and caffeine, all of his symptoms of depression left!

Hormones can affect your brain. I've found that an imbalance of estrogen in a woman and testosterone in a man can cause brain fog, the lack of the ability to concentrate and depression. Dr. John Lee confirms this link in his July, 2001 *Medical Letter* where he wrote that estrogen decreases thyroid function, based on an article in the *New England Journal of Medicine*.[30] For that reason, I recommend that you see your natural healthcare professional for help balancing your hormones. Also, read my book on hormones called, *Why Am I So Wacky?*

When Janice came to see me, she was taking many drugs, including several anti-depressants and she told me at the end of the appointment, that if I hadn't given her some answers, she was going to commit suicide that day! I put Janet on a transdermal progesterone cream before she left my office. Within three days, she sent me flowers, saying how much better she felt and that her crying had stopped. Within two weeks she was back to work, after struggling for the past year! She's still doing well with the nutritional changes and supplements I recommended.

I've had a male client who wanted to use progesterone as well. His comment was, "I had no temptation to be depressed. It was dramatic and quick. Don't take me off it!"

Certainly there are appropriate times for anti-depressants. A doctor has to diagnose clinical depression and they can recommend this type of help for a severely, depressed person going through difficult times.

Here's a test for depression from the American Psychiatric Association.[31]

1. Do you have a poor appetite with weight loss or increased appetite and weight gain?
2. Do you have insomnia or increased need for sleep?
3. Are you agitated or hyperactive, or do nothing all day?
4. Do you have a loss of interest or pleasure in usual activities and a decrease in sex drive?
5. Do you have fatigue and loss of energy?
6. Do you have feelings of worthlessness, self-reproach, or inappropriate guilt?
7. Do you have diminished ability to think or concentrate?
8. Do you have recurrent thoughts of death or suicide, or suicide attempts?

If you answered yes to most of these questions, see your doctor. But realize even if you are diagnosed with major depression, there are nutritional deficiencies involved, and without addressing these, you may perpetuate your depression.

Low Thyroid and Depression

After my client, Cathy, had her thyroid oblated through nuclear medicine (her doctors gave no other option for treating her diagnosed Grave's disease) she was supposed to remain on thyroid replacement hormones for life.

She sought my help because she still struggled with fatigue, depression and weight gain. Her health profile pointed to Chronic Fatigue Syndrome. Twelve months later, using whole-food supplements and modified eating habits, she no longer struggled with fatigue and depression. Her weight gain stopped, and she finally began to lose weight. She's been completely medication free for ten months.

Martin Budd, a D.O. and author of *Why Am I So Tired?,* explores the relationship between the thyroid and many diseases. In his book, he says that if you suffer from low grade hypothyroidism your entire body can feel mentally and physically depressed. He believes it's vital to determine whether you have low-grade hypothyroidism in order to effectively treat depression. **He also writes that depression occurs as a result of physiological, not psychological disfunction.** Depression is now largely seen as a nutritional or biochemical disorder.[32]

Synthroid is one of the top-selling drugs for the thyroid. Yet according to Dr. John Lee, the FDA has chastised the manufacturer of the drug, as having a product that can't be considered safe and effective. Yet it's been on the market for 40 years![33] The closest things to natural, safe thyroid supplements are Armour, Westhroid and Naturethroid.

Dr. Schwarzbein considers synthetic thyroid hormone a stimulant because it increases serotonin to the brain. However, stimulants eventually deplete serotonin. So often, however, someone on thyroid hormone is now prescribed an anti-depressant to increase serotonin. She considers the problem one of malnutrition, not low-thyroid.[34]

This epidemic reflects our American lifestyle of fast food eating and lack of exercise. Like I've always said, "You can't solve a nutritional problem with a drug." And as a weight-loss counselor, I've discovered that many anti-depressants cause weight gain. This makes people even more depressed! So anti-depressants often just handle the symptom of depression; they never get to the cause.

The Link Between B Complex and Depression

Jessica was helped tremendously with the B complex. Here are her comments:

> I spent years on anti-depressants. It can take 2-3 weeks for the anti-depressant to have any positive effect. After my visit with Lorrie, I felt better instantly, and progressively better in the next 24 hours. Why would anyone go on an anti-depressant when they can take B vitamins?

There are definite links between nutritional deficiencies and depression. Unfortunately, most teenagers live on junk foods and diet cokes or beverages loaded with caffeine. Not only do these foods and beverages cause B vitamin deficiencies, but in addition, teens rarely eat foods with the B vitamins. Our attitude, memory, clarity and emotional states all depend on having sufficient B vitamins.

You can get B vitamins from eating eggs, nuts, seeds and meat. However, stress, caffeine, poor digestion and junk food often interfere with the absorption of these vitamins.

Early signs of B complex deficiency are characterized by depression. Serious B deficiency symptoms are: anxiety, hostility, emotional instability, craving for sweets, mental confusion, and irritability.

Ritalin and Depression

According to researcher Dr. Bruce West, Ritalin is now the drug of choice for children and adults with Attention Deficit Disorder (ADD). More than four million children take this drug. Yet Ritalin causes many side effects, including lethargy, depression and suicidal tendencies. He adds that examining many school shooting cases, these children were on this type of drug therapy or under psychiatric therapy.[35]

The sad thing about the prescription of Ritalin is that no one is looking for the cause of the depression or hyperactivity. They are simply using the drug to mask symptoms of an underlying health or nutritional problem.

In her book, *The ADD Nutrition Solution,* Marcia Zimmerman says that Ritalin or other stimulants do nothing to cure or correct the problems that are causing AD/HD. In the years between 1990 and 1997, overall sales revenues for Ritalin increased 600 percent to about $450 million annually. She adds that stimulants and anti-depressants are not harmless drugs, but heavy-duty controlled substances.[36] **Most children simply have low-serotonin levels from their high sugar diet.** Her book recommends the vitamin B complex and Omega 3 fats.

Prozac, Zoloft and other anti-depressant drugs prescribed can cause side effects including nausea, vomiting, headaches and fatigue! What's the point?

I've helped these children with proper nutrition, supplements, and eliminating all stimulants. Many children taking Ritalin who are labeled "slow learners" or "lazy," aren't necessarily lazy by nature. Some have just been extremely malnourished. One client I've helped reported that not only does her child not fall asleep in class, but he's even improved his grades from Ds and Fs to As and Bs!

More Help for Depression

Depression caused by a chemical imbalance, such as low serotonin levels, can be helped with diet. Drugs and stimulants such as caffeine, tobacco and alcohol accelerate thyroid activity, but then later depress thyroid function. Following the dietary guidelines in Part 5 of this book will help your body make normal serotonin levels.

While St. John's Wort has been used for thousands of years, it is medically approved for the treatment of depression, anxiety and insomnia in Germany. Sales there outnumber all other anti-depressants. If you decide you want to try St. John's Wort, do not take it while you are already taking an anti-depressant. (See your natural health care professional or Clinical Nutritionist for more help.)

If you are hypothyroid, (low thyroid) how can you assure that your thyroid gland will function normally so you can lose weight? See a natural health professional who can recommend a natural thyroid hormone supplement. He or she may additionally recommend supplements for better thyroid function. Also, according to Dr. Wilson, if you have both thyroid and adrenal stress, you may need nutritional support for the hypothalamus, which will help both glands.[37]

Scientific research shows that Omega 3 Fatty Acids help the brain with mood and memory. Omega 3 fats are found in fish and flaxseed. Dr. John Lee says that women who eat Omega 3 fish while pregnant decrease their chances of developing postpartum depression.[38]

Nutrition for Depression

Taking the antioxidant vitamins A, C, E and the mineral selenium are great. Bioflavonoid antioxidants found in berries and carotenoid antioxidants such as orange, yellow and red fruits and vegetables are great. You can get these foods in your diet by including blueberries on your cereal, an orange for breakfast, and carrots and tomatoes in a salad for lunch.

Ginkgo has been extensively studied for its ability to improve circulation and memory support. Kava has had a long history of safe use for depression. However, misleading reports in Europe made health professionals cautious in using Kava. Initially, concern over 29 cases of possible liver damage was reported in Germany and Switzerland. According to Dr. Lee, what was omitted from the report was that in 21 cases, pharmaceutical drugs linked to liver damage were also involved.[39]

Recommended supplements for low thyroid:

·Iodine or kelp

·Selenium and Magnesium

·Vitamin B complex

·Essential oils (Omega 3 fats)

·Desiccated Thyroid Supplement

·Antioxidants

Recommended supplements for depression:

·Vitamin B complex and Folic acid/B12

·Essential oils (Omega 3 fats)

·Ginkgo

·St. John's Wort

·Probiotics and liver detox

Let's move on to blood-sugar levels and fatigue.

Chapter Four

Why Am I Always Tired and Hungry?

Clients often come in complaining of unexplained fatigue. We commonly think this is just old age. So here is my definition of old age: You know you're getting older when it takes more time to recover than it did to wear you out!

If we've already ruled out adrenal or thyroid fatigue, my nutritional testing and questions often indicate something that may be quite easy to fix: imbalanced blood-sugar levels.

It's hard to "feel good" with low blood-sugar levels! As a motivational speaker, I always include nutritional advice in my speeches because it's impossible to stay "positive" when your unbalanced body chemistry is working against it!

Recently, a male musician came to see me regarding his fatigue. After a few visits, we discovered he had a sluggish thyroid, and that he was eating too much refined white sugar. He explained to me that growing up, it was common for them to have a dessert after every meal. The idea that there was anything wrong with sugar seemed impossible.

Regarding his work, he said,

> I felt so guilty. I wasn't doing as much as I needed to. I was thinking maybe I was lazy. I had to force myself to get out of bed. I never imagined that I would feel so much better by just changing my diet and balancing my blood-sugar levels.

What about you? Let's just look at a few questions to see if you have low-blood sugar.

Nutrition Test #4

1. Do you frequently crave sweets or carbohydrates?
2. Do you get dizzy and weak if you miss a meal?
3. Do you feel irritable or depressed throughout the day?
4. Do you have frequent thirst?
5. Do you have heart palpitations?
6. Do you have dark circles under your eyes?
7. Do you seem overly emotional?
8. Do you get headaches?
9. Do you have unexplained fatigue?
10. Do you have a family history of hypoglycemia or diabetes?

If you have three or more of these symptoms, you may have some type of blood-sugar problem. However, these questions can be tricky. So often when I ask my clients if they crave sugar, they automatically reply, "No." Later, however, they may tell me that they drink coffee with sugar, soda, or even alcohol daily. No wonder they don't crave sugar after already taking in so much of these sugar-filled substances!

Today diabetes is on the increase, with an estimated 17 million Americans diagnosed every year. It's guessed that nearly 5 million Americans have undiagnosed diabetes. And hypoglycemia (low-blood sugar) is also on the rise, even among young children. Symptoms include fatigue after eating, irritability, sweet cravings, and hunger. If not controlled, it can lead to serious medical complications, such as heart disease, stroke, kidney failure, high-blood pressure, amputations resulting from damage to nerves and blindness.

Symptoms of Low-Blood Sugar

- Fatigue
- Cravings
- Heart problems
- Dizziness
- Headaches
- Depression
- Irritability if meals are missed
- Rapid heart beat
- Inability to concentrate
- Low body temperature
- Blurred vision
- Weakness
- Weight gain

What's the major cause of low-blood sugar and the resulting condition of fatigue? Refined sugar! Other causes are a poor diet of processed starches combined with chronic stress and lack of exercise. The good news is that eating well can help the pancreas, adrenal, liver, thyroid and every other part of your body!

High-Insulin Levels and Fat

Symptoms of shaking, sweating, and experiencing a rapid heart beat are often linked to the adrenal glands which also play a part in blood-sugar control and high-insulin levels. Dr. John Lee says that when insulin is chronically high, once your cells have all the glucose (sugar) they can handle, most of what you eat will turn directly to fat. Years ago, Nobel Prize winner Linus Pauling argued that it wasn't the fat that was the culprit in weight gain, it was the refined carbohydrates.[40]

When insulin levels are high, so are "bad" LDL cholesterol levels and triglycerides. Insulin also causes the kidneys to retain water and salt, which raises blood pressure. High-insulin levels are linked to imbalances in hormone-like biochemicals called, eicosanoids, that control blood pressure, blood clotting, inflammation, and pain sensations. High-insulin levels are also linked to many types of cancer.[41]

You need to understand the source of the information you read. For example, I've read diabetic literature that highly promoted fat-free products, all of which raise your insulin! Also promoted are non-caloric sweeteners, such as Nutrasweet, which are linked to brain damage, cell damage and weight gain. I encourage my diabetic clients to eat a low-carbohydrate diet, and to use the herb, Stevia, as a sweetener.

Sugar Makes Us Tired

Dr. Nancy Appleton, author of *Lick the Sugar Habit,* lists nearly eighty scientific references that show how sugar makes us not only tired, but also sick.[42]

In addition to throwing off the body's homeostasis, excess sugar may result in a number of other significant consequences. The following is her list of some of sugar's metabolic consequences from a variety of medical journals and other scientific publications. I have acquired permission to publish her list because I think it's so very important to understand that **sugar is at the root of our fatigue, as well as most degenerative diseases.** (Her web page is www.nancyappleton.com.)

What Else Does Sugar Do?

1. Sugar can suppress the immune system.
2. Sugar can upset the body's mineral balance.
3. Sugar can cause hyperactivity, anxiety, concentration difficulties, and crankiness in children.
4. Sugar can cause drowsiness and decreased activity in children.
5. Sugar can adversely affect children's school grades.
6. Sugar can produce a significant rise in triglycerides.
7. Sugar contributes to a weakened defense against bacterial infection.
8. Sugar can cause kidney damage.
9. Sugar can reduce helpful high-density cholesterol (HDLs).
10. Sugar can promote an elevation of harmful cholesterol (LDLs).
11. Sugar may lead to chromium deficiency.
12. Sugar can cause copper deficiency.
13. Sugar interferes with absorption of calcium and magnesium.
14. Sugar may lead to cancer of the breast, ovaries, prostate, and rectum.
15. Sugar can cause colon cancer, with an increased risk in women.
16. Sugar can be a risk factor in gall bladder cancer.
17. Sugar can increase fasting levels of blood glucose.
18. Sugar can weaken eyesight.
19. Sugar raises the level of a neurotransmitter called serotonin, which can narrow blood vessels.
20. Sugar can cause hypoglycemia.
21. Sugar can produce an acidic stomach.

22. Sugar can raise adrenaline levels in children.
23. Sugar can increase the risk of coronary heart disease.
24. Sugar can speed the aging process, causing wrinkles and grey hair.
25. Sugar can lead to alcoholism.
26. Sugar can promote tooth decay.
27. Sugar can contribute to weight gain and obesity.
28. High intake of sugar increases the risk of Crohn's disease and ulcerative colitis.
29. Sugar can cause a raw, inflamed intestinal tract in persons with gastric or duodenal ulcers.
30. Sugar can cause arthritis.
31. Sugar can cause asthma.
32. Sugar can cause candidiasis (yeast infection).
33. Sugar can lead to the formation of gallstones.
34. Sugar can lead to the formation of kidney stones.
35. Sugar can cause ischemic heart disease.
36. Sugar can cause appendicitis.
37. Sugar can exacerbate the symptoms of multiple sclerosis.
38. Sugar can indirectly cause hemorrhoids.
39. Sugar can cause varicose veins.
40. Sugar can elevate glucose and insulin responses in oral contraception users.
41. Sugar can lead to periodontal disease.
42. Sugar can contribute to osteoporosis.
43. Sugar contributes to saliva acidity.
44. Sugar can cause a decrease in insulin sensitivity.
45. Sugar leads to decreased glucose tolerance.
46. Sugar can decrease growth hormone.
47. Sugar can increase total cholesterol.
48. Sugar can increase systolic blood pressure.
49. Sugar can change the structure of protein causing interference with protein absorption.
50. Sugar causes food allergies.
51. Sugar can contribute to diabetes.
52. Sugar can cause toxemia during pregnancy.

53. Sugar can contribute to eczema in children.
54. Sugar can cause cardiovascular disease.
55. Sugar can impair the structure of DNA.
56. Sugar can cause cataracts.
57. Sugar can cause emphysema.
58. Sugar can cause atherosclerosis.
59. Sugar can cause free radical formation in the bloodstream.
60. Sugar lowers the enzymes' ability to function.
61. Sugar can cause loss of tissue elasticity and function.
62. Sugar can cause liver cells to divide, increasing the size of the liver.
63. Sugar can increase the amount of fat in the liver.
64. Sugar can increase kidney size and produce pathological changes in the kidney.
65. Sugar can overstress the pancreas, causing damage.
66. Sugar can increase the body's fluid retention.
67. Sugar can cause constipation.
68. Sugar can cause myopia (nearsightedness).
69. Sugar can compromise the lining of the capillaries.
70. Sugar can cause hypertension.
71. Sugar can cause headaches, including migraines.
72. Sugar can cause an increase in delta, alpha and theta brain waves, which can alter the mind's ability to think clearly.
73. Sugar can cause depression.
74. Sugar can increase insulin responses in those consuming high-sugar diets compared to low sugar diets.
75. Sugar increases bacterial fermentation in the colon.
76. Sugar can cause hormonal imbalance.
77. Sugar can increase blood platelet adhesiveness which increases risk of blood clots.
78. Sugar increases the risk of Alzheimer's disease.

You and I may have grown up eating refined white sugar, but did you know that chemically refined white sugar is fairly recent? According to Mary June Parks in *A New You,* for centuries, sugar was sold by the teaspoonful only through drug stores. Originally crude, unrefined beet sugar was a luxury. Sugar was served on rare occasions or used as a medicine for the treatment of gout.[43]

In Ann Louise Gittleman's book, *Get the Sugar Out,* she reports that sugar consumption has increased tremendously in the U.S. We eat between 170 to 200 pounds of sugar per person, per year. Our body was not designed to eat refined white sugar. In the 1800s, people ate between 12 to 25 pounds of sugar per person, per year. As the rate of sugar consumption has increased, so has the rate of diabetes.[44]

Other Links to Diabetes

Dr. Bruce West reports several links to diabetes.

> Diabetes is linked to processed foods and tap water. Processed foods are saturated with synthetic sugars, such as glucose, dextrose, corn syrup, corn sweeteners, high dextrose corn syrup, and other similar names. They are made from corn, but produced synthetically. They are a danger to human health and were originally banned in the U.S. and Canada. In 1906, the first head of the FDA tried to ban glucose and artificial sweeteners because they cause diabetes in animals. Since industry runs this country and the government, he failed. The sweeteners have been with us ever since and are the basis for the epidemic numbers of folks with diabetes.[45]

He adds that what's even worse is the combination of glucose or artificial sweeteners and the chlorine and chloramines from chlorinated tap and shower water. Chlorine makes the sweeteners even more harmful, increasing their power to induce diabetes.[46] (In case you take showers while drinking diet pop! Seriously, though, research like this helps us to investigate all of the possible causes of such serious diseases.).

Dr. Earl Mindell, author of *Prescription Alternatives,* says that if you have adult onset diabetes and your physician isn't working with you to aggressively treat the disease with diet and exercise, then you are being shunted into a money-making pipeline for the medical industry. He believes that the majority of Type II diabetes, especially when it is caught early, can be very successfully treated with diet, exercise and supplements.[47]

Dr. Bruce West also says that Type II diabetes is mostly caused by diet and lack of exercise. In his practice more than 80% of all Type II diabetics can get off medication or insulin with the proper diet and exercise. And even the Type I diabetics can dramatically reduce their need for insulin given proper diet, supplements, and exercise.[48]

Recently, I saw an ad for Zocor, a cholesterol lowering drug which stated, "Surprisingly, 7 out of 10 people with diabetes also have high cholesterol."

Surprisingly? If you have diabetes, your cholesterol is also high because improper handling of sugar is related to high cholesterol. So in addition to all of the diabetic drugs you are already taking, now you can take another one: Zocor. According to the patient statement, some side effects can include hepatitis, jaundice, fatty changes in the liver, and, rarely, severe liver damage and failure, cirrhosis, and liver cancer. Zocor also interferes with normal fat metabolism.

A safer approach is to change your diet and exercise!

I recommend Ann Louise Gittleman's book, *Get the Sugar Out* for 501 ways to cut the sugar out of your diet, including breakfast, lunch, dinner, snacks, treats, eating out, and even getting it out of your mind!

What Can I Do?

If you lack energy and suspect you have hypoglycemia or diabetes, have your doctor run a glucose tolerance test. Eliminate high-sugar foods, refined processed foods, such as instant rice and potatoes, pasta, white flour, sodas and alcohol. Be sure to get enough essential fatty acids from flaxseed oil or fish such as salmon. Eat foods lower on the glycemic scale (See Chapter 11 for more specifics on the glycemic index, meal planning and nutritional supplements.)

Craving sugar isn't natural, and there is always a reason. Perhaps you don't eat enough protein meals. Or you may be eating too many processed carbohydrates, or not eating enough of the essential fats. You may have a chromium, zinc, or magnesium deficiency since all three minerals are related to the handling of sugar in your body. Magnesium is great for chocolate cravings as well. (I use a Standard Process chromium product with my clients called Cataplex GTF which is only sold through certified health professionals.)

Additionally, the herb Gymnema helps the body to handle insulin levels and helps eliminate sugar and carbohydrate cravings.

Take a vitamin B complex supplement. Dr. Bruce West in his article in "Disease and Prevention" says that thousands of people with hypoglycemia are really suffering from a B-Complex deficiency called B Complex Deficiency Syndrome (BCDS).[49] Only pure, natural food-based supplements will overcome this deficiency. But this supplement isn't as effective if you keep eating starches and sugars! The B complex vitamins are vital for carbohydrate metabolism. Also, take the antioxidant vitamins A, C, E and selenium in a whole-food supplement form.

Recommended supplements:

·Chromium GTF and Zinc

·Vitamin B complex

·Essential oils (Omega 3 fats)

·Magnesium (chocolate cravings)

·Antioxidants (vitamins A, C, E and selenium)

·Gymnema

Exercise is also vital for keeping your blood sugar level. You'll learn more about that in Chapter 10.

Let's continue to understand why we are so tired, but often unable to get the sleep we need.

PART FOUR

Why Am I So Sleepy?

Chapter Five

Why Can't I Sleep?

I find that when couples come to see me, to properly help the insomniac, it's important to get the whole story. Sometimes the one who is sleeping all night keeps the other one awake simply by their outrageously loud snoring!

Even though often overlooked, we desperately need enough sleep for good health. Lack of sleep could be the main reason for fatigue. It's hard to stay healthy without adequate sleep! The human growth hormone is released during your sleep to help repair bones and muscle. Your adrenals, liver and thyroid all regenerate during restful sleep.

Many people are plagued with various types of insomnia. Some can't sleep at all while others sleep too much. Or some people get to sleep, but wake up in the middle of the night, often around 3:00 a.m., unable to return back to sound sleep.

Some people have sleep apnea, which involves a series of interrupted sleep cycles all night. Some people have blocked passageways in their nose which could be corrected with surgery. Other people might be overweight which could cause sleep apnea. I've had hundreds of clients with sleep problems, and like energy problems, they are varied. In order to help people with Chronic Fatigue Syndrome or Fibromyalgia, it's vital to help them get the sleep they need.

We'll look at more detail about how to get to sleep in Chapter 10, but first let's look at the role of sleep and sleep medications.

Are Drugs Your Final Answer?

Taking drugs is so common today. If you can't sleep, you might buy a common over-the-counter sleep aid, such as

Sominex® or Extra Strength Tylenol PM®, or your doctor might give you a prescription for a sleep aid.

We are so used to going to the doctor to get a pill to fix something. Maybe it's medication for insomnia, maybe it's for headaches, allergies, or high-blood pressure. Why do we spend billions of dollars a year on health, yet never get over the problem? In many cases, people are encouraged to use these medications forever.

So many sleep problems are really lifestyle problems. However, how often have you heard your doctor say, "I think you need to change your diet and lifestyle." More commonly he says, "Take this sleeping pill." There are times that drugs may be helpful, but they treat the symptom and only provide symptomatic relief. They are not without side effects.

Let's take a common sleep aid, Ambien®, for example. According to Dr. Earl Mindell, in clinical trials of this drug, 4 to 6 percent of subjects stopped taking Ambien® because they were so bothered by the side effects. These included headaches, dizziness, lethargy, depression, anxiety, runny nose, and urinary tract infections.[50] It should only be used for 7 to 10 days, but how many people do you know who only take a drug for a week? Most of my clients didn't even know about the side effects.

Drugs May Cause Fatigue

Did you know that most drugs make you tired? Drugs rob energy from the body and change the body's priorities to focus on the drug, but the cause of the problem is not eliminated. People are still sick, and now they have to stay on drugs a lifetime to stay symptom-free, often having to increase the dose and/or change medications in an attempt to remain symptom-free as they become worse.

Side effects, which result when drugs are administered, are the body's effort to eliminate the drug. For example, if a skin rash develops after taking a medication, this is the body's effort at pushing this toxic substance out of the body.

Medications are necessary at times for life-threatening situations, but drugs are ultimately not solving the problem—we are not sick due to medication deficiencies. In fact, any drug given to a healthy person will make him sick, due to its toxic effect. Yet the doctor gives the same drugs to a sick person and expects him to get well! **How can a body be poisoned back to health?**

Healing never happens with drug therapy. Many of our "diseases" for which we need drugs were really caused by poor lifestyle combined with a poor diet.

Finding the Cause

Following a poor diet for many years can contribute to sleep problems. For example, most people who have come to me with this problem tell me that they, at one time, used to drink several bottles of soda a day, or they used to eat a lot of sugar or processed carbohydrates. Eventually, these habits caught up with them. Often sleep problems are just another variation of severe blood-sugar imbalances. My first goal is to help them with their diet to maintain normal blood-sugar balance, following the principles in Part 5 of this book.

Drinking too much caffeine or soda a short time before bed is another common cause for a sleepless night, but so is anything else stimulating such as exercising late at night, or experiencing great emotional stress.

Obviously, if a person continually stays up too late, they can throw off their normal sleep cycles. I help them make lifestyle changes so that they can get to sleep earlier.

Another cause of insomnia is severe thyroid or adrenal fatigue. According to an article in the *Journal of Clinical Endocrinology and Metabolism,* overactive adrenals lead to insomnia. Investigators monitored the sleep of 11 patients with insomnia and 13 people without sleep disturbances. They found that their adrenal hormone levels were significantly higher in the insomniacs than the control group. They also found that increased production of stress hormones is likely to lead not only to depression, but also to high-blood pressure, obesity and osteoporosis.[51]

Obviously when a person is fatigued, getting enough sleep is so important. But more importantly, not getting enough sleep can cause even more serious problems. According to the Annual Meeting of the American Diabetes Association, chronic lack of sleep may cause people to become less sensitive to insulin. Over time, this can raise the risk of obesity, high-blood pressure and diabetes. They report that sleep loss is a risk factor for Type II diabetes.[52]

Another article in the *Journal of the American Medical Association* (JAMA) reported that sleep problems may have an adverse impact on these diseases: Parkinson's disease, Alzheimer's disease, Multiple sclerosis, kidney disease, GI tract disorders and behavioral problems in children.[53]

Finally, too little sleep may accelerate aging. According to an article in *Lancet,* only getting a few hours of sleep can hinder metabolism and hormone production in a way that is similar to the effects of aging.[54]

I help the client change their diet by eliminating stimulants such as caffeine and sugar. When appropriate, exercise helps insomniacs tremendously! These people are often low in the entire B and C complex, as well as minerals such as magnesium and calcium which help them sleep. Herbs such as Valerian Root and St. John's Wort are helpful as well. Another key step is to follow a liver detoxification program. This is thoroughly explained in my book, *Why Do I Feel So Lousy?*

Recommended supplements:

·Calcium and/or magnesium

·Zinc, chromium and gymnema

·Vitamin B and C complex

·Essential oils (Omega 3 fats)

·Valerian Root or St. John's Wort

·Liver detoxification program

Also, see Part 5 for help in diet and lifestyle changes. If you have a serious sleep problem, I would suggest a sleep clinic. Let's now look at the relationship between digestion and fatigue.

Chapter Six

Why Does Poor Digestion Cause Fatigue?

We often take digestion for granted. I recently had a gentlemen tell me his digestion was fine. When I saw his paperwork, I noticed that his digestion was his biggest complaint. When I asked him about it he said, "Oh, I am a little constipated, I have stomachaches a lot and have a little gas, but isn't that normal?"

No, it's not normal, but it is common! We were designed for good digestion and good health. In working with people with Fibromyalgia and Chronic Fatigue Syndrome, **I've found that most energy problems involve digestive problems.** A good example is at Thanksgiving. People eat a huge meal, and they then need to take a three-hour nap!

Americans pop digestive aids like candy and spend millions of dollars a year on laxatives and antacids; yet they continue to suffer from poor digestion and elimination. If these products really "fixed" the problem, why do we still need these drugs? What's the real problem? In his book, *The Mysterious Cause of Illness,* Dr. Jonn Matsen explains that our stomachs "harden" in response to eating and drinking certain substances.[55] We then think we can eat anything, because we seem to get away with it for a time. Sooner or later, however, digestive problems surface. This is the beginning of fatigue and even disease.

Ideally, we should not only have good digestion, but we shouldn't even get sick. Here's why. Our first defense against foreign invaders is the stomach where hydrochloric acid (HCl) kills germs. Enzymes in the gastrointestinal tract are also designed to assault these germs. If people lack enzymes and HCl, they will have poor digestion. But more importantly, germs that would have otherwise been killed are allowed through the digestive tract.

Did you know that we are bombarded by toxins inside and outside the body? Our second defense is the liver which is incredible at breaking down and eliminating these toxins. However, sugar and processed foods impair the liver's ability to break down and eliminate toxins.

And finally, our gastrointestinal tract is lined with "good" bacteria which influence our health. More than 400 of these microorganisms, which collectively weigh about 3 pounds, should inhabit our digestive tract. Unfortunately, the average American only has about one pound of this "good" bacteria.

This "good" bacteria fights against "bad" bacteria, viruses, fungus and other disease-producing microbes. They are also important because they synthesize B vitamins and aid in the digestion of fiber. Without these good bacteria, "bad" bacteria grow out of control. When that happens, the body can suffer many symptoms.

What About Antibiotics?

Discovering antibiotics in the 1930s was a breakthrough for modern medicine but is such a common practice today that the body is building a resistance to them.

The term "antibiotic" literally means "against life," and is a substance that inhibits growth or kills living organisms, in most cases, bacteria. One of the problems with antibiotics, however, is they do not differentiate between the bad bacteria which cause harm and the good bacteria found normally in the body.

We all have good bacteria to help proper digestion and assimilation of food and to keep other naturally occurring organisms such as yeast and fungus in check. When an antibiotic is taken, it attacks **all** susceptible organisms including the good bacteria causing a gap in the digestive process and leaving other organisms to take over. This is why all antibiotics can cause diarrhea or constipation and can lead to thrush or yeast infections. The longer the course of treatment, the more likely a person will experience side effects. These include: fatigue, gastrointestinal upsets, Candidiasis, severe skin rashes, kidney and renal infections, diarrhea, colitis, hearing loss and many more. (For more detail on Candida and health, see my book, *Why Can't I Lose Weight?*)

I always advise caution when considering the use of antibiotics. They should only be used for bacterial infections, and only for short-term therapy.

Nearly every client I have seen with CFS has had a history of long-term antibiotic treatment. William G. Crook, author of *Chronic Fatigue Syndrome and the Yeast Connection* concludes that the **overuse of antibiotics is a major contributing factor to the developing of yeast infections and chronic fatigue.**[56]

More About Side Effects

Certainly the most common side effect of antibiotics is the varied yeast infections that occur when antibiotics kill the good bacteria. For that reason people must take "probiotics," or "friendly bacteria," for at least two weeks to replenish their good bacteria.

According to Dr. Don Colbert, when antibiotics throw off your proper balance, the bad bacteria grow like a wild fire out of control with nothing to slow them down or stop them. Now your body is in trouble, because the bad bacteria may produce toxins which weaken your immune system.[57]

In his book, *Peak Immunity,* Luc De Schepper writes,

> Although acute viral infections like influenza kill thousands of people each year...most people are able to defeat these tiny invaders. Other viruses have a different approach. Between attacks, they will lie dormant in the body, waiting like vultures to reactivate in moments when the host's immune system is suppressed.[58]

According to author Earl Mindell, 98 percent of infections would have gotten better with some very basic care, such as rest and fluids. Yet we think antibiotics will cure everything from cholera to a hangnail. American physicians write 40,510,000 prescriptions for antibiotics every week![59]

We, however, have taken them so often that many common strains of dangerous bacteria have become resistant to antibiotics, making the drugs all but useless.

Another problem is the practice of adding antibiotics to livestock feed in the meat and dairy industry to prevent infection caused by the substandard living conditions of these animals. According to Dr. John Lee, not only has this exposed Americans to small amounts of antibiotics on a regular basis, it has created even more strains of resistant bacteria.

In his *John Lee Medical Letter*, Dr. Lee reports that 20 percent of ground meat in supermarkets is contaminated with dangerous bacteria, half or more of which is resistant to antibiotics. The risk is highest for those whose immune systems or digestive systems are weak.[60]

New generations of bacteria can quickly become resistant to our drugs so drug companies have to develop newer, better antibiotics. Dr. Richard Krause, of the National Institute of Health, said in an article published in *Science Magazine* that doctors in hospitals around the world are losing the battle against an onslaught of new drug-resistant bacterial infections. This includes staph, pneumonia, strep, tuberculosis, dysentery, and other diseases that are difficult, if not impossible, to treat.[61]

According to Dr. Michael Schmidt, antibiotics kill the good bacteria in the gut and impair the immune system, making the condition worse. He believes that using antibiotics causes increased susceptibility to intestinal infection by fungi, bacteria, viruses and parasites because the antibiotics alter this balance of intestinal organisms.[62]

Not All Drugs Are Safe!

People commonly take many drugs and yet are often oblivious to their side effects. For example, Accutane® is commonly prescribed to teenage girls for acne, in spite of the fact that it has been known for years that it can cause birth defects. According to the Centers for Disease Control (CDC), Accutane® continues to cause birth defects even though teens taking it are supposed to have two pregnancy tests a month.

Dr. Lee says, "Since the drug company can't protect teens from getting pregnant while taking this drug, and since there are many other ways to control acne these days, isn't it time to take this danerous product off the market?[63]

Researcher Dr. Bruce West reports that medical drugs are the fourth leading cause of death in America today.[64]

What Can We Do?

To eliminate fatigue caused by improper digestion, take a digestive enzyme with hydrochloric acid. Also, replace the good bacteria destroyed by antibiotics through the use of probiotics. The most common probiotics are acidophilus and bifidus usually available in health food stores. They also are in yogurt, but look for the "live yogurt cultures." Take probiotics any time antibiotics are prescribed and for several days after. They can be taken on a regular basis to maintain healthy digestion with less constipation and bloating.

Seek the help of your natural health care professional who can provide nutrients that strengthen the immune system.

Tired people are also toxic. I encourage my clients to do some type of "internal" cleanse twice a year. (I use a product sold only through health professionals called Standard Process Purification Program. See my book, *Why Do I Feel So Lousy?* for additional information.)

Recommended supplements:

·Digestive enzymes

·Probiotics

·Vitamin B complex

·Essential oils

·Fiber

Let's move to Part 5 to understand how to live a healthy, energy-producing lifestyle.

PART FIVE

Designing Your Life for Energy

Chapter Seven

What Should I Eat?

What if we had to determine the guidelines for eating healthy by looking at fast-food restaurants? We would probably conclude that the "basic food groups" are: French fries, burgers, sodas and ice cream!

We've looked at why we are tired. Now let's see how eating the right kinds of foods is one of the best ways to help you regain the energy you desire and keep your health. Remember the foods you eat affect your energy, your life and your success!

Are You Confused?

From working with thousands of clients, what I've seen is that until someone has some type of health problem, most people just eat what their parents ate, or whatever is fast, convenient and tastes good. They assume that if it's sold at a grocery store or restaurant, it must be good for them.

I remember thinking that way before I changed my diet in the mid '70s. We are bombarded with misinformation primarily due to the interests of the food and drug industries who attempt to get you to buy whatever they are advertising.

Author and Certified Nutritionist Carol Simontacchi says it this way:

> Over the past century, the American food culture has gone through a transformation so pervasive and enormous that we have almost completely lost sight of what constitutes a normal diet.[65]

The largest manufacturing industry in America is processed foods, and industry influences research studies.

According to researcher Sally Fallon, universities have powerful ties to the food processing industry. She cites Dr. Frederick Stare, from the nutrition department at Harvard University as a good example. Early on, he wrote several articles implicating vegetable oils—not animal fats—as one of the major causes of heart disease. After he became department head, the university received several grants from the food processing industries. After that, his articles said that there was nothing wrong with white bread, sugar and processed foods. He even suggested Coca-Cola as a snack food![66]

If you browse on almost any nutritional bookshelf, you'll find book after book implicating saturated fats as the cause of heart disease. Most heart-healthy cookbooks still follow the "low-fat" lifestyle, recommending recipes loaded with refined sugar and processed white flour. We are encouraged to eat margarine instead of butter and millions of people have eliminated red meat from their diet. So even though Americans have decreased the amount of saturated fat in their diets for the last 20 years, heart disease has more than doubled. Why? Because these are just a few bits of misinformation that the public commonly accepts as facts.

We're Getting Sicker!

Cancer and heart disease were rare at the turn of the century. Today one in three people will die of cancer and one in two will die of heart disease. We have epidemics of chronic fatigue, digestive problems, diabetes, and learning disabilities which were rare in the 1900s.

In his foreword to Dr. Robert Arnot's book, *The Breast Cancer Prevention Diet,* Dr. Michael P. Osborne says, "We know that the most important environmental factor in the cause of breast cancer is nutrition." He says that we could wait for results of scientific studies which will be available years from now, or use the information we now have that suggests a potentially effective nutritional preventive strategy. This includes eating real, whole foods that prevent cancer as well as fight cancer.[67]

A *New York Times* article written by Marion Burros explains that the American Dietetic Association (ADA) takes the "wishy-washy stance" that there are not "good or bad foods," because they rely on food industry money which "means that they never criticize the food industry." The ADA is funded by food companies.[68]

Think about the cholesterol issue. While most of the information you hear concentrates on issues of cholesterol in foods, according to an article written by Sally Fallon in *Consumers' Research* magazine, nutritionists have known for years that heart disease is linked to processed foods, including white sugar, soft drinks, white flour and synthetic vitamins.[69]

Even as far back as the 1940's, Dr. Royal Lee said:

> America's food industry is built to a large extent on foods which would ordinarily be highly perishable. Rather than finding methods of efficient distribution, it has been easier to simply devitalize the food. Foods which have had their vital factors removed will fail to sustain life for insects, molds, and microbes; consequently they can be easily shipped over long distances, and simply stored over long periods. Unfortunately foods which will not sustain other forms of life, will not satisfactorily sustain human life.[70]

The surprising thing is that junk foods are so pervasive! A friend named Chris recently went on a mission's trip to Brazil. She was impressed that there weren't any overweight people. Throughout the 12 days that she was there, she lost 12 pounds without even trying! I asked her what she thought the reason was, and she said that there was no junk food around! In America, we're surrounded with junk food. Help!

For a long time I've thought that it might help if we label foods according to what they do. For example, "sleep-inducing" donuts, or "artery-clogging" sandwich spreads. That might motivate us to make "healthy" choices!

Let's look at various types of foods and how they make us tired.

How Sugar Makes Us Tired

Most people think that a candy bar will give them energy, so from an early age, they associate eating foods with sugar as energy-producing foods. What really happens is that they cause fatigue. When you eat sugar, you feel a temporary lift. Then the body floods the bloodstream with insulin and other hormones to lower the blood-sugar levels and bring them back to normal levels. Too much insulin becomes toxic to the body. Time after time, as you eat more and more sugar, the processes that normalize our blood-sugar levels begin to wear out. Eventually, the blood sugar levels stay either lower or higher than normal. Too much insulin causes high cholesterol, high triglycerides, high-blood pressure and even clogged arteries. According to Dr. Diana Schwarzbein, sixty percent of heart disease is caused by high-insulin levels.[71]

What else causes high-insulin levels? Stress, dieting, caffeine, alcohol, aspartame (as in NutraSweet), lack of exercise, drugs, eating a diet deficient in protein and fat, and eating excess carbohydrates.[72]

If continued long enough, other conditions can manifest including obesity, depression, heart problems, learning problems, and symptoms common to a diabetic. As our consumption of sugar has increased, so has our rate of heart disease. We weren't designed to eat refined white sugar, and as I mentioned earlier in this book, we only ate about 12 pounds per person, per year in the 1820s. Today, people eat upwards of 200 pounds per person, per year.

Sugar causes many deficiencies. I explained in my weight-loss book that during the processing of raw sugar cane, most of the nutrients, including the B vitamins and minerals are completely removed, and chemicals are added. Your body pulls from your own store of B vitamins every time you eat white sugar. So eating white sugar, or foods which contain white sugar makes you tired, which doesn't help your energy crisis![73]

Sugar is so toxic, that getting a stomachache after eating sugar is a real, natural response. But we override it by giving our children a little sugar every day, to where our digestive system eventually says, "I give up." Your stomach stops sending obvious messages like nausea or vomiting. Instead, it just gets more and more irritated. Later on, we "develop" symptoms like allergies and autoimmune diseases or leaky gut and digestive problems. I'm not surprised at how many children and parents have eliminated allergies and/or skin problems when they eliminated sugar from their diet.

Sweet, Healthy Alternatives to Sugar

Common alternatives to sugar include raw honey, raw maple syrup, molasses and barley malt. Crystallized raw cane juice, otherwise known as Sucanat, looks like brown sugar, but has more nutrients. Stevia is a natural South American herb that is very sweet, but does not cause an insulin response. Xylitol has recently received a lot of press. It's an extract that looks and tastes like sugar. It's also slower to cause an insulin response and may help prevent cavities.

But it's not easy for people to change. When my mother read about sugar and the evils of eating sugar, she gave up reading!

How Carbohydrates Make Us Tired

Processed starches turn to sugar quickly in the liver. That's why white flour and white-flour products also make us tired. Some examples of white flour products are: white bagels, white breads, white muffins, white cake, cookies, and snack foods such as donuts and Twinkies®.

Did you know that up to 70 percent of the essential nutrients are lost in the production of white flour? In the refinement process, more than 21 nutrients are taken out, and only a handful are put back in and what is put back is synthetic. There is so much evidence of the correlation between heart disease and white flour that Dr. Lee said, **"We might as well remove the term heart disease and supplant it with 'white-flour disease.'"**[74]

Eating processed carbohydrates also raises your insulin levels. Insulin is a fat-storing hormone. Glucagon is a fat-burning hormone which is released when we eat proteins. Our goal is to release more glucagon for more stable blood-sugar levels and weight loss, and lower insulin levels.

Serotonin is our "feel good" neurotransmitter. We may not always consciously recognize it, but one of our goals for eating is to keep our serotonin levels high.

Eating processed carbohydrates (and stimulants) raises our insulin levels, which raises our serotonin levels. That is why people feel emotionally good after eating chocolate and foods made with refined sugar. Unfortunately, if we continually raise our insulin levels by eating processed carbohydrates and processed sugar, our serotonin levels fall too fast. So we will want to eat more carbohydrates or sugar, to create more serotonin. Eventually, we become fatigued and possibly now depressed. The reason we are craving these stimulants is that we became low in serotonin.

It's become common for people to go to their doctor with this condition, and more often than not, the doctor gives them Prozac® or some anti-depressant. However, we aren't deficient in Prozac®! Anti-depressants are a bandaid remedy; they never get to the cause of the problem which is stimulants, or substances that overstimulate the body. In fact, often anti-depressants never even help. Our goal, though, is to have normal blood-sugar levels so we make insulin properly, and finally make normal levels of serotonin.

The U.S.D.A. Food Pyramid, which recommends 6-11 servings of carbohydrates can easily provide 250-500 grams of carbohydrates a day. No where in history has man eaten that many carbohydrates! We have more stress in one day on our pancreas than our ancestors had in their entire lifetime!

Can Vegetarians Be Healthy?

When I was a compulsive overeater, and 40 plus pounds overweight, I was also a vegetarian. I was teaching cooking classes, while I ground whole-grain kernels to make whole-grain breads. Clearly, the vegetarian diet that contains high amounts of carbohydrates, such as pasta, bread, and cereals can contribute to high insulin, low-serotonin levels. Most vegetarians I've worked with are also depressed due to this. Really, I wasn't a vegetarian; I was a "Pastaterian!"

Diets high in starches, fats and sugars all raise insulin levels. We'll look at how to choose the right carbohydrates in the next Chapter.

How Stimulants Make Us Tired

After you drink caffeine, it causes stress to your heart and adrenal glands. This creates high levels of cortisol which not only burn out your adrenal glands, but also further cause abdominal obesity and disease.

Most of the people that I see who complain of being fatigued usually drink some type of caffeinated beverage: coffee, tea, sodas or sugared drinks.

That's because **all** stimulants—sugar, coffee, caffeinated beverages, and alcohol—affect your serotonin levels in the brain. After the quick burst of energy, they raise your insulin levels which eventually deplete your serotonin levels again. However, as your serotonin levels fall, you need more of a stimulant. So you go for **more** sugar, or more caffeine. Then, these stimulants overstimulate the adrenals again, and eventually you become tired again. This is how addictions develop. We need to break this cycle! We can break the cycle with a proper diet and whole-food supplementation.

How Fats Make Us Tired

Fats give us energy. So why would fats make us tired?

"Bad" fats are processed fats. They can make us tired because they are so indigestible. These bad fats include vegetable oils which were damaged in processing with high temperatures or chemicals, and hydrogenated and partially-hydrogenated oils, such as margarine and Crisco. In the hydrogenation process, hydrogen molecules are added to a good vegetable oil which damages the fat and also makes it saturated. These damaged fats, also known as "trans fats," are linked to free radical damage, heart disease and cancer.

For many years, I read articles about how butter was a "saturated" fat and we shouldn't eat it if we were trying to lose weight, or if we had high cholesterol. According to health researcher Paul Addis, cholesterol is **not** the cause of heart disease but actually is an antioxidant against free radicals in the blood, and a repair substance that helps heal arterial damage. He explains that as with fats, cholesterol may be damaged by exposure to heat and oxygen. Damaged or oxidized cholesterol is what promotes injury to the arterial cells.[75]

Where can you find oxidized or damaged cholesterol? In powdered eggs, fried foods, and fats processed with high temperatures. Again, damaged fats are called trans fats.

More On Cholesterol

But did you know that eighty percent of cholesterol is produced by the body itself?

According to author Diana Schwarzbein, the fear of cholesterol from fat is not grounded in science. Fats don't **cause** heart disease, and on the contrary, the more "good" fat you eat, the healthier you become.

She explains that cholesterol is vital to the body. It's a precursor to hormones such as progesterone, testosterone, and estradiol. We need good fat for the brain, as well as for good health. Fats don't stimulate the insulin response.[76]

When you restrict dietary cholesterol you force the body to make its own cholesterol. That's when your body makes **more** cholesterol than it needs. So when you eat a meal without cholesterol, your body overproduces it. So you can have high cholesterol levels from eating high-insulin foods! Because insulin is the major hormone directing the overproduction of cholesterol in the body, lowering insulin levels and eating more cholesterol are two of the best things you can do to lower cholesterol levels.[77]

So the best way to lower cholesterol levels is not to restrict dietary cholesterol, but to stop the process by which cholesterol is made. Eat a diet low in sugars and processed carbohydrates. Read labels, throw away margarine, and eliminate all deep-fried foods. Eat good fats such as olive oil, and include the Omega 3 fats that are found in cold-water fish such as salmon and tuna.

Butter Is Better!

Dr. Royal Lee considered raw, unpasteurized butter to be one of the highest values in food products obtainable. In one of his reports, he wrote, "Butter is rich in vitamins A, D, E and F. Taken the year round, butter contains enough vitamin D to be considered a preferred source of this vitamin."[78]

In this same report, Dr. Lee even quoted a study that simply used butter to treat psoriasis, xerophthalmia [a skin disease], tuberculosis, dental caries and rickets![79]

He also said that substituting vegetable oils for butter caused a decalcification of bones, resulting in their fragility, which he believed was a vitamin F deficiency.[80]

What about all of these hydrogenated "fake" butters that don't melt and taste awful? Butter is better. Hydrogenation is great for preserving the food, but not for preserving us! If the food you are considering buying starts with the phrase, "I can't believe it's...." you probably can believe that it's not a real food! I can't believe that people still buy these foods!

What about salt? It's interesting that a salt deficiency can actually be as dangerous as excess salt. The issue about salt is again about processing. The table salt most people use is highly refined, having been treated with many harmful additives, including aluminum compounds. Even dextrose is added to salt, and finally, bleach. (See *Why Can't I Lose Weight?* for more information on salt alternatives.)[81] Unprocessed sea salt is rich in minerals, and is the best to use.

What About Fruits and Vegetables?

We've looked at the dangers of processed sugar, processed carbohydrates and processed fats. What about processed fruits and vegetables?

There are so many studies on the benefits of "five-a-day," for preventing disease, that entire books have been written about them. As with the case above, however, we need real fruits and vegetables, not processed ones. This means we should eat the whole piece of fruit, such as an apple or orange, rather than drink apple juice or orange juice. For many people, drinking juices eventually floods their body with insulin, again making them tired. It's better to eat fresh than frozen, although frozen is preferred over canned vegetables.

Without these real, whole foods, our cells become damaged, our glands become tired, and the process of aging begins.

What Should I Eat?

Our goal is to eat regular, balanced meals of unprocessed protein, fats and carbohydrates from real whole foods. We need to eat enough protein, fat and carbohydrates to keep our blood-sugar levels normal so we won't crave stimulants. And we need to eat to feed the liver, adrenal and thyroid, the major energy-producing glands. When we eat balanced meals, (as outlined in Chapter 11), we will naturally produce enough serotonin, which keeps us happy and healthy.

Next, let's review my Ten Life Design Principles for Energy.

Chapter Eight

Ten Life Design Principles for Energy

My clients like knowing that there are real causes for their fatigue. They tell me that it's terrible to wake up and feel so tired in the morning, when they didn't even stay out late the night before!

My goal with every client is to help them change their lifestyles so they can have more energy. Here are ten principles that I published in my weight-loss book, *Why Can't I Lose Weight?*, that apply as well for energy.[82]

Principle 1: Support Your Digestion

Nearly everyone needs some support for their stomach, colon, and liver. By improving digestion and especially helping the liver, energy is improved. Most of my clients have felt better and gained more energy by taking digestive enzymes, doing a colon cleanse, and supporting their liver. (You can learn more about these in my book, *Why Do I Feel So Lousy?* See my book list at the back of this book.)

Principle 2: Drink Pure Water

Drink plenty of reverse osmosis purified or distilled water, (not tap water) at least 1/2 your body weight in ounces daily. For example, if you weigh 100 pounds, drink 50 ounces of pure water. Your body is 75-85 percent water, and you need it to flush out toxins. Did you know you can become dehydrated by drinking coffee, juice, sodas and even herbal tea? Your body wants water! I recommend putting lemon or lime slices in your water for even better digestion, if you can handle citrus fruits.

Though you can drink less water if you eat plenty of high-water content fruits and vegetables, most people don't get enough of either.

Principle 3: Eat Light at Night

Have you ever skipped meals all day, only to make up for it by eating a huge dinner and several snacks at night? How did you feel the next day? Sluggish? I used to do that and it always made me feel tired and gain weight!

Try not to skip meals, especially breakfast. To keep your blood-sugar level normal, try to start your day with something for breakfast—even if it's a protein drink or fruit with nuts.

Also, try not to eat after 8:00 p.m. You'll have more energy if you eat the majority of your calories earlier in the day.

Principle 4: Eat Healthy Snacks

Your snacks should be protein-fat combinations such as peanut butter with celery or cheese with a whole-grain cracker.

I used to give my clients a day off where they could eat whatever they wanted, but we found this idea worked against them. The refined, white sugar and processed foods set up another cycle of binges and cravings. This added two more days before they would lose weight!

We were born with a natural sweet tooth that can be satisfied by eating fresh or dried fruits which combine well with almonds. Occasionally, make "special treats" with healthy ingredients. (See my *Why Can't I Lose Weight Cookbook?* for ideas.) Be encouraged. After three to six months of no refined sugar foods, you may notice that you don't even like the taste, and it won't be so hard to resist.

Principle 5: Eat More Fruits and Vegetables and Limit the Bread and Pasta

One of the most important principles for energy is to build your meals around healthy vegetables. Most of us eat salads for lunch only on occasion. We'll have a side order of cabbage slaw with a burger or a carrot salad at the deli. But salads are wonderful-as long as you don't overwhelm them with a high-fat dressing! In a balanced diet of carbohydrates, protein, and fat, vegetables and fruits are your energy-producing staples!

Vegetables and fruits are alkalizing to the body. Simply put, it means that we don't become overly acidic, a condition that can also lead to fatigue.

Eating more servings of fruits and vegetables will increase your vitamin, mineral, and enzyme intake, especially those important antioxidant vitamins: A, C, and E. For example, one apple provides 1500 mg. of vitamin C. Eat colorful vegetables. Rather than eating a white potato, have sweet potatoes or yams for a good healthy change. Easily-digestible fruits and vegetables help keep your energy up and your appetite down.

The average American eats about 200 grams of carbohydrates a day, and most of them are processed. (The stuff we really want, such as pasta, breads and cereals!) As I've already said, eating too many carbohydrates (especially the processed ones) depletes, rather than gives us energy.

I recommend you eat fewer carbohydrates (three 1/2 cup servings a day) and when you do eat them, eat the complex carbohydrates. These include: Oatmeal, barley, brown rice, millet, rye, spelt, and small amounts of wheat products if there is no allergy to wheat.

The best way to lower high-insulin levels and gain more energy is by limiting the amount of "high-glycemic" foods you eat. The Glycemic Index is determined by how much sugar or glucose each food contains on a scale from 0 to 100. Foods low on the index such as green vegetables, cause a small rise in blood sugar after they are eaten. Foods with a high glycemic index, such as white bread or pasta cause a higher rise in blood sugar.

For energy and weight loss, choose foods with a low glycemic index.

Generally, fruits, vegetables and whole grains are lower in sugar than their processed counterparts. You may want to use the sample Glycemic Index in Chapter 11 (page 104) to help you choose energy producing foods.

You can find a more detailed Glycemic Index chart at your local bookstore, but a good rule of thumb is that the more natural and whole a food, the less slowly it will turn to sugar in the body (which can make you fat and tired!)

In the last chapter, I recommended that you eat the whole piece of fruit, such as an orange, rather than drink the orange juice. Oranges have a lower glycemic index than the juice. Generally, fruits, vegetables, lean protein, and complex carbohydrates all are lower on the Glycemic Index.

Principle 6: Eat the Right Fat

Eat essential fatty acids in the form of extra-virgin olive oil, salmon, tuna, almonds, or take a supplement of evening primrose oil or flaxseed oil. These oils are required by our body and we must get them from foods. They are vital for energy, weight loss, healthy digestion, and proper hormone functioning. Avoid products with hydrogenated oils (peanut butter, margarine, Crisco), all fried foods, and processed vegetable oils, and anything with trans fats. Limit saturated fat in the form of red meat.

When shopping for oils be sure they are 1) cold-pressed, 2) refrigerated, and 3) come in dark bottles. Otherwise, they may be rancid or spoiled. For example sunlight or any light that gets through clear bottles depletes nutrients in oils.

Principle 7: Eat High-Quality Protein

It's vital that you balance your meals with protein, fats, and carbohydrates. If you don't get enough protein, you may begin to crave sugars and carbohydrates. However, if you don't get enough carbohydrates you won't have the building materials for serotonin production. And we need the right types of fat to feed your brain, your glands, and to help prevent cravings.

Vegetarian protein can be helpful and effective. Used moderately, beans and legumes can be good sources of protein and fiber. Black beans, lentils and kidney beans are easy to use in recipes and are good for diabetics.

Protein drinks and meal replacement bars can be great supplements, if they aren't high in carbohydrates and natural or refined sugars! The best protein drinks are nondenatured whey protein. Read labels; some of them are extremely high in sugar! They should be 6 or less grams of carbohydrates and no sugar. (I sell several healthy, low-carbohydrate products made by Standard Process, which is only sold through health professionals.)

Drinking a protein drink once a day is a healthy lifestyle change; however, drinking them too often may be counter-productive, unless you are following a clinical cleanse. Eventually, you will crave foods that you can chew!

Principle 8: Drink Caffeine-Free Beverages

I recommend that "lemon water" be your drink of choice. Squeeze 1/4 of a lemon in 8 ounces of water and sweeten with a dash of the herb, Stevia. Avoid coffee, soft drinks, black tea and chocolate, which all contain caffeine. Caffeine depletes the body of the B and C vitamins, and some minerals. Caffeine is implicated in anxiety, PMS and mood swings.

Principle 9: Stay Motivated

It's hard to get or stay motivated when you are exhausted! As you've already seen in this book, fatigue can come from nutritional deficiencies, hypothyroid (low thyroid) or hypoadrenal (low adrenal).

Every day I recommend changes in people's diets that can prevent these imbalances so they feel like exercising! See the list of recommended nutritional supplements in Chapter 11.

Some estrogen hormone products, for example, encourage weight gain, fatigue and depression. You will need to see your doctor or qualified nutritionist for these.

Additionally, we have to face the facts about sugar, processed carbohydrates and bad fats. They don't give us energy! But giving up foods that we like can be hard. We have to convince ourselves that the benefits of receiving energy and health are worth making changes, and that we would rather give up the instant pleasure for long-term gain.

One tip is to substitute healthier alternatives for the unhealthy foods. For example, why not eat an apple instead of a cookie? (For more help with motivation, read my book, *Why Can't I Stay Motivated?*)

Principle 10: Get Regular Exercise

Exercise is vital for health and energy. But doesn't it seem logical that if someone is tired, they don't find exercise particularly appealing? Who wants to exercise if they can't get out of bed? I recommend that you handle your energy crisis; then exercise. (See Chapter 10.)

Chapter Nine

What Vitamins Do I Need?

Nearly everyone in America has taken some type of vitamin or mineral at some time in their life. Funny how we all end up with a collection. I did, before I learned some important differences between vitamins. Here's how we get them. We'll watch a TV infomercial about a specific product, or read a magazine and run out and get the latest supplement for something. Later though, we forget what we have and why we bought them in the first place!

We've just looked at processed foods and how they are one of the main reasons that we are tired. But they are also one of the main reasons for vitamin deficiencies.

Do We Really Need Supplements?

Often, I'm asked "If we ate better, could we get everything we need from food?" No!

There has never been a study of the American diet proving that we get all the vitamins and minerals we need for optimal health through our food. On the contrary, you can pick up almost any issue of the *American Journal of Clinical Nutrition* and find study after study citing nutritional deficiencies that are linked to heart disease, cancer, diabetes, and so on.

Never before have we eaten so many refined and processed foods with so many missing nutrients. Never before have we been exposed to so many chemicals. And never before have we experienced so much stress and fatigue.

Maybe there was a time when we did get everything from food. One hundred years ago, many people lived on farms and ate their vegetables which were plentiful.

Not today. Some surveys indicate that as many as 59% of our calories come from nutrient-poor foods such as soft drinks, white bread, and snack foods. Our foods don't contain as many nutrients as they once did.

In 1941, in an attempt to prevent disease, the Food and Nutrition Board of the National Research Council prepared guidelines for vitamins and minerals called the Recommended Dietary Allowances (RDAs). They were originally set up to reduce the rates of serious nutrient-related deaths from diseases such as scurvy, which is a vitamin C deficiency, beriberi, from a lack of thiamine or vitamin B1, and pellagra, a deficiency of niacin, or vitamin B3.

The old RDAs were never designed to prevent cancer; they just prevented the above-mentioned deficiencies. While we need 10 milligrams of vitamin C to prevent scurvy, we need more than that to prevent heart disease. But it's not easy to get it. A U.S.D.A. government survey of 21,500 people found that not one single person consumed 100% of the RDAs, from the foods they ate. We need to deal with these nutritional deficiencies. Let's look at some.

Iron Deficiency Anemia

Iron is related to energy production because red blood cells need iron in order to deliver oxygen throughout the body. Symptoms of iron deficiency anemia include fatigue, weakness, fainting spells, pale skin, shortness of breath, and heart palpitations.

Iron is essential for energy production and a healthy immune system. Anemias can mean a reduction in the number of red blood cells, or reduction in the size of red blood cells. In these cases, red blood cells are deficient in hemoglobin, the iron-containing portion of the blood which helps oxygenate the blood. Pregnancy and lactation are two times when women need iron supplementation. When a woman has a hormone imbalance or she cannot metabolize calcium, (the two main causes for excess bleeding, as with longer or heavy menstrual cycles), this can also induce anemia.

While iron deficiency anemia is the most common, there are many types of anemia. Anemia can be caused by deficiencies of B6, B12, folic acid or copper.

The most common cause of iron deficiency is chronic bleeding or a diet low in iron, high in phosphorus (sodas), poor digestion, ulcers, or excessive caffeine consumption.

Often low iron and B12 indicates too little stomach acid. **So taking hydrochloric acid helps you absorb iron.** (I use Standard Process Zypan for this.) Eat more iron rich foods, such as red meat and other animal protein such as eggs, fish, poultry, green leafy vegetables, dark raisins, and blackstrap molasses. Iron absorption is enhanced by taking it with vitamin C. Phosphorus, which is found in most soft drinks hinders iron absorption. Taking calcium can inhibit the absorption of iron, so take calcium supplements at bedtime.

If iron deficiency is due to excess bleeding, this may be an indication of hypothyroid or hormone imbalance. Check these with your natural health care professional or Clinical Nutritionist.

You may get too much iron because it's stored in the liver, spleen, bone marrow and blood. Too much iron leads to the production of free radicals (this is linked to heart disease) and increases the need for vitamin E. Check with your health care professional or Clinical Nutritionist before supplementing with iron. The serum ferritin test and transferrin saturation test can tell if you have too much stored iron.

Pernicious Anemia and B12

Pernicious anemia is commonly defined as anemia from impaired intestinal absorption of vitamin B12.

Symptoms of pernicious anemia include fatigue, pale color, numbness in fingers and toes, heart palpitations, diarrhea, a sore, red swollen tongue, and senility.

B12 is absorbed in the stomach and small intestine. A protein produced in the gastrointestinal tract called the intrinsic factor combines with chemicals in the intestine to make B12 available to the body. Low levels of this factor also cause low blood levels of B12. Additionally, some types of stomach problems, such as gastritis can cause low levels of the intrinsic factor. Taking an enzyme with hydrochloric acid, (such as Zypan by Standard Process), enhances absorption.

B12 helps folic acid in regulating the formation of red blood cells. Strict vegetarians need to take B12 supplements, as this vitamin is found mostly in animal foods. The best sources of B12 are eggs, liver, brewer's yeast, mackerel, milk and dairy products.

Folic Acid Deficiency

A deficiency of folic acid can also cause anemia. Folic acid is vital for red blood cell formation and is commonly known to prevent birth defects. Recently, much research shows that Folic acid helps combat depression, anxiety and the treatment of cervical dysplasia. Folic acid works best when combined with B12.

Folic acid is vital for regulating homocysteine levels. High levels of homocysteine can damage your coronary arteries. Just taking Folic acid with B12 can prevent this. Many people feel Folic acid and the B complex are important nutrients for preventing high cholesterol and heart disease.

Folic acid is important for pregnant women since it helps with fetal nerve cell formation.

Signs of Folic acid deficiency include fatigue, anemia, digestive disturbances, weakness, and shortness of breath. The best sources of Folic acid are brewer's yeast, green leafy vegetables, beef, chicken, and fish. The birth control pill can increase the need for Folic acid.

Let's Check Your B's

Fatigue can be the result of simply not getting enough nutrition. For example, the B vitamins found in breads, cereals and beans are essential for energy. They are natural energy boosters, and this water-soluble vitamin is the most common nutritional deficiency in America. The B complex helps with symptoms of fatigue, low energy, low immunity, lack of mental power, and stress overload. Memory loss, emotional instability and reduced attention span are linked to B vitamin deficiencies.

As I said earlier in this book, it is possible to get your B vitamins from a perfectly balanced diet. It's also possible to get into Macaroni Grill or TGIF on a Friday night without any line, but the chances of either are slim! In our society, stress and a poor diet make this almost impossible. Caffeine, sugar, alcohol, and tobacco rob the body of B vitamins.

So take a B complex supplement. I recommend one made from whole foods, rather than synthetic.

Vitamins A, C, E and selenium are considered antioxidant vitamins and are also vital for energy production. A good whole food vitamin supplement will contain them all. But be wary of ones with names like “A Buncha Vitamins” or “Almost All the Vitamins You Probably Need!" (I explain how to purchase vitamins in my book, *Why Do I Need Whole Food Supplements?*)

How About Your Minerals?

Minerals are important too. American soils are dangerously low in these minerals which are catalysts for vitamin usage. Other minerals, such as zinc, are crucial for energy and proper immune function.

Chromium deficiency can also cause energy depletion, which is why chromium is sold as a weight loss and energy supplement. Chromium is involved in the metabolism of glucose. It helps maintain stable blood sugar levels and helps both diabetics and hypoglycemics. Our American diet is low in chromium due to lack of it in our soil and the overprocessing of foods. Chromium deficiency leads to anxiety, fatigue, and blood sugar problems. Food sources of chromium include brewer's yeast, whole grains, blackstrap molasses and liver.

Get the whole form, chromium GTF, or the glucose tolerance factor, which is extremely effective. Diabetics who take a chromium supplement should discuss it with their physician since their insulin requirements will decrease.

Magnesium helps manufacture ATP energy for cells by assisting calcium and potassium uptake. Magnesium is even more important to prevent heart disease than calcium and it helps prevent cardiovascular disease. Magnesium deficiency symptoms include insomnia, rapid heartbeat or palpitations, hypertension, chronic pain or fatigue and chocolate cravings.

Magnesium is found in fish, meat, dairy and seafood, blackstrap molasses, brewer's yeast, green leafy vegetables, and sesame seeds.

It's not natural to have to take food supplements, but unfortunately, our American soil is dangerously low in so many minerals, that we simply can't get the nutrition from just food any more. Most people need at least a multiple vitamin and mineral supplement. I highly recommend whole-food supplements such as the ones I use in my office made by Standard Process. (Again, for more information on why we need supplements and how to buy them, see my book, *Why Do I Need Whole Food Supplements?* which is listed on the last page of this book)

Chapter Ten

How Should I Live?

We Americans are funny. We often live in the fast food lane year after year, neglecting our health, and then when we are sick and tired, we wonder what went wrong!

It's amazing how Americans can spend so much time on other things: their jobs, making money, taking care of the children; and yet neglect the one most important thing that needs to be taken care of: their bodies. Yet everyone knows when the body suffers, everything else suffers—the job, relationships, and the ability to make money.

Real energy comes from a well-nourished body! To be healthy we also need enough rest, to lower our stress and to have regular exercise. Let's start with sleep.

Get a Good Night's Sleep

In her book, *Potatoes Not Prozac,* Kathleen DesMaisons recommends that you eat a small snack that contains a protein and carbohydrate before bed. This helps stabilize your blood-sugar levels Low-blood sugar or hypoglycemia can cause you to wake up at night.

The high-sugar or high carbohydrate diet contributes to insomnia because it crowds out the foods we need to produce the good hormones that help us sleep. These foods include eggs and yes, even butter! Good fats, proteins and small amounts of carbohydrates help the body to maintain balanced insulin levels which further create balanced serotonin levels and finally the proper conversion to melatonin.

Tips For Getting a Good Night's Sleep

When you sleep is as important as how long you sleep. Here are some additional tips for sleep problems.

1. Try to get to sleep between 10:00 to 11:00 p.m. If you stay up until 1:00 or 2:00 in the morning, it only further exhausts your adrenals, even though that may be an energizing time of day for you. It would be ideal if you could sleep in past 7:00 in the morning, but this isn't always possible. Getting to bed too late can wear out your adrenals.

Taking a 20-minute nap when you feel tired is like a vitamin pill for your adrenals! So if you need a nap, don't feel guilty about taking it, but when you become healthier, you won't need these naps.

2. One of the best cures for insomnia is adding regular exercise to your life. You don't have to run a marathon, but make it vigorous enough that you sweat.

However, don't exercise late at night unless you know your levels of cortisol. If your cortisol levels are too low, you may sleep better when you exercise at night because exercise raises cortisol. If your cortisol levels are too high, you will want to relax before going to bed. (You can have your health professional or Clinical Nutritionist order a saliva cortisol test to determine if your levels are too high or too low.)

3. Eliminate caffeine and caffeinated products. Caffeine causes your store of neurotransmitters to be depleted which may make you feel perpetually exhausted without it. I help my clients wean off caffeine while simultaneously restoring their adrenal health. Eventually, they no longer need the stimulants and their sleep cycles are restored.

4. Try not to eat large meals (or snacks!) right before bed. It's best not to eat later than 7:00 or 8:00 at night so your body can work on digesting the foods before you sleep.

5. Eliminate alcohol which can cause interrupted sleep patterns and makes you wake up between 3:00 and 4:00 a.m.

6. Try herbs such as Kava or Valerian Root or minerals such as calcium or magnesium. (See Chapter 2 on adrenal stress.) I don't recommend melatonin supplements. A better way to produce melatonin is to try to get 15-30 minutes of sunlight in the day, and keep your room dark at night. I use a wonderful supplement called Min-tran which has helped hundreds of people. Also, take a nice hot bath before bed.

7. Avoid sugar and processed carbs before bed, which will raise your blood-sugar levels and cause you to wake up in the middle of the night. Follow the recommendations in Chapter 11 of this book.

8. Try not to watch stimulating TV shows or read a suspense novel which would wind you up before going to bed. Read something that would relax you.

Stress Management

In Chapter 2, I discussed stress as a source of fatigue, so stress plays a big role in health. Eating well, getting enough sleep and exercise are important, but so is handling stress.

It's impossible to live stress-free, but there are many things we can do to help our bodies handle stress.

For many people who have been burning the candle at both ends for so long, it's going to take more than a weekend to recover. For some clients, it's taken 6 months to a year. But don't put off the recovery process because your adrenals won't heal on their own.

1. Stay well nourished. Many stress management programs I've seen tell you to "calm your mind." You can't have a calm mind if you are guzzling coffee and sodas! Taking the B complex vitamins is vital for stress management. I recommend that the first change you make is in your diet following the suggestions in this book, including the supplements listed for adrenal health in Chapter 2 and Chapter 11. Herbs which help with relaxation and sleep also help with stress. The best are Valerian Root, Kava and St. John's Wort.

2. Set goals for a healthier lifestyle, being realistic about your life and what you can do. I believe in time management because if we don't nail down important appointments, our time gets away from us. I've written an entire book on goal setting and time management including tips that help me enjoy a healthy lifestyle and even manage my time so that I have been able to have an effective writing schedule. Following that schedule has helped me to write eight books, so I know it was effective for me. (For information on *Why Can't I Stay Motivated?* see the back page of this book.)

3. Schedule regular times for recreation. When I first started writing, I didn't know how to pace myself. I can work long hours at a time, so I did. I didn't even realize how much I needed to get away and play, until I became burned out and depressed. I was fortunate to have several friends who literally came and took me out! Now I have learned how to pace myself; I write about 6 hours a day on the weekend instead of 12-14; and I spend time with friends and recreation. I'm more productive when I get back to work. I recommend mini-vacations or light hobbies.

4. Examine your life and beliefs. Recently I was listening to a tape by a teacher named Joyce Meyer. The tape was entitled, "No Worries," which is a common phrase in Australia. Joyce was saying that while in Australia, they were rushing to get to the meeting where she was speaking. She frantically asked, "Are we going to make it?" The Australian hosts said, "No worries!" She might have only been a few minutes late, but as she said, she had a choice. She could either be stressed over it or just relax. She couldn't help the situation, but she did have some control over how she reacted to the stress.

There will always be something to worry about: your job, economy and relationships. But most of the things that we get upset about don't matter. Worry is stress and it can even make you physically sick.

Amanda, one of my clients said, "I've learned to stop the chatter in my mind when I feel a panic attack come on. I say to myself I know I am feeling this now, but if I let it ride, it will be better. I will be okay. I've had to talk myself out of stress and panic."

Amanda also said that she had more problems with panic attacks when she was eating a poor diet and processed foods. So changing her diet and her mind both have helped her to manage stressful situations.

I have a helpful exercise I use when I get under stress. I write down my thoughts on paper such as, "What's the worse thing that could happen? What can I do about it?" Often just seeing the situation on paper helped me to bring it into perspective. And if I truly had done everything I knew to do, then there really wasn't anything else to do but have faith and confidence that it will all work out. It's amazing how often things just work out.

5. Relax and take time out for a 15 minute "quiet time." When I get to work, the phone rings, and I see clients most of the day, and even sometimes during the lunch hour. I know that if I don't take time before work, I won't have any time to myself to just think and to put things into perspective. The early morning is when I like to pray and read my Bible which builds my faith as well. But you might prefer to have some time at night, when your chores are done and everyone is in bed. It helps us all to have time where we don't have to do anything, or be anywhere. I'm so surprised at how parents go everywhere, nearly every night of the week. I encourage clients to sit down and really prioritize all of these activities. Does your child have to be in every activity?

I'm sensitive to women, because I find they are the ones who are tending to the needs of everyone else in the family, while their needs often go unmet. While they may not see this as anything serious, over a long period of time, this can cause stress and illness. Everyone needs a break every now and then. If you are a husband, I think getting your wife a day at the spa once in awhile is really great! At least, take her out to dinner or have a date night once a month. It will do wonders for both of you.

There are many books written on prayer, meditation and relaxation. Recently, one of the bath stores at our local mall had a gift set which included bath salts and gel, a relaxing CD and a book on doing nothing! I found it to be a great gift! Taking a warm bath with lavender or lemon grass helps relax the muscles. There are many healing aromas to choose from.

A natural way to raise melatonin levels is to soak in a hot bath for 20 minutes. That is much healthier than taking a melatonin supplement for sleep, because long-term use can lead to a further, imbalanced biochemistry.

6. Laugh more! People take life so seriously, and that's okay to a point. I try to make life fun with humor, whether it's with my friends or clients. Laughter is healing. Just the act of smiling changes chemicals in your brain. Rent a funny movie or read funny books. These habits will keep your serotonin levels naturally high.

Energy-Producing Exercise

You say you're too tired to exercise? I understand. After being nutritionally tested for adrenal and thyroid function, following a healthy eating plan, and taking your whole-food supplements, you will have more energy.

Starting an exercise program is like changing your diet. You have to start slow, one day at a time. But sometimes things motivate us. I had to put training wheels on my treadmill. Or noticing that our knees buckle but our belt won't. Or you hear "snap, crackle and pop," but you aren't eating anything! One client's idea of weight lifting was just getting off the couch. I still think that if God had meant for us to touch our toes, he would have moved them up the leg!

I want to encourage you to start where you are. So many people set unrealistic goals for themselves, only to fail. Set a goal for 15 minutes of activity, for example. That way you can begin a consistent exercise program. As you feel better, you will be able to increase your time.

Be careful to eat well when you exercise. Studies show that exercise produces much acid, so it's important that you eat plenty of fruits and vegetables. Excess acid is linked to fatigue, stomach problems and even diseases such as gout.

I believe we are more motivated to do things for ourselves when we know the benefits. Besides getting more energy, another great benefit of regular exercise is that it helps reverse insulin resistance. In other words, it helps your body handle insulin properly so you can finally lose weight, gain more energy and produce more of the important serotonin.

So, here are 55 benefits to regular exercise to help you convince yourself that it's good for you and worth your time. Exercise helps you(r):

1. Improve your breathing.
2. Improve your circulation.
3. Improve your muscle tone.
4. Decrease your weight.
5. Relieve stress.
6. Spend less time feeling sick.
7. Sleep better.
8. Feel more confident with higher self-esteem and self-worth.
9. Feel more in control of your body.
10. Be more active and productive.
11. Enjoy life with a better attitude.
12. Have more control of your life.
13. Extend your chances of living longer.
14. Have clearer nasal passages.
15. Skin look more supple.
16. Ability to burn fat to be more efficient and increase your metabolism.
17. Replace fat with lean tissue; you will lower body fat and lose inches.
18. Combat depression.
19. Lower your blood pressure.
20. Improve your coordination and balance.
21. Normalize/lower your blood sugar.

22. Increase oxygen to the brain which makes you more alert and clear thinking.
23. Decrease your appetite.
24. Increase overall flexibility.
25. Improve your ability to fight disease because your immune system is strengthened.
26. Lower your set point.
27. Reduce the risks of heart disease.
28. Increase the chance of surviving a heart attack and stroke.
29. Reduce fatigue and increase strength.
30. Improve your posture.
31. Reduce chances of developing varicose veins.
32. Relieve and/or prevent constipation.
33. Decrease your desire for nicotine and other substances.
34. Burn calories more consistently.
35. Strengthen your bones/helps prevent osteoporosis.
36. Remove lactic acid and other poisons from the body.
37. Slow down the aging process.
38. Enjoy a better sex life.
39. Increase your chances of being self-motivated.
40. Improve your relationships.
41. Prevent senility.
42. Achieve lifetime weight control.
43. Increase your HDL cholesterol.
44. Decrease your cancer risk.
45. Improve diabetes management.
46. Lower your resting heart rate.
47. Improve your work performance.
48. Reduce lower back pain.
49. Improve stress management.
50. Reduce anxiety.
51. Increase endurance.
52. Improve your vision.
53. Cleanse the body of toxins.
54. Absolutely improve the overall quality of your life.
55. Have an avenue for a healthy means of escape.

Oxygen Gives You Energy

The number-one killer in the United States is cardiovascular disease. Eating a healthy diet is vital to prevent heart disease, but it's also vital to work the heart muscle to get oxygen to the tissues.

Aerobic means "with oxygen." Aerobic exercise means you make a certain amount of demand on your body that is strong enough to get your heartbeat to 70 percent of your maximum heart rate. Additionally, aerobic exercise reduces insulin secretion and increases glucagon secretion, the hormone for fat-burning. And from what we have said about carbohydrates and insulin, it's not a good idea to load up on carbohydrates before aerobic exercise.

The best types of aerobic exercise are: running, walking, jogging, swimming, inline skating, racquetball, cycling, rowing, ice-skating, tennis, speedwalking, cross-country skiing, aerobic dancing, jazzercize, stair-climbing, skiing, and using a stationary bike or mini trampoline.

Anaerobic exercise, like weight resistance training, helps the body to release one of the best fat burners there is, the human growth hormone. Therefore, combining both aerobic and anaerobic exercise can lower fat and increase lean muscle mass.

To stay at your current level of fitness, exercise three days a week. To improve your fitness, exercise four to six days a week. You need to take a day off every week for your body to rest and recuperate.

How To Start An Exercise Program

Note: Before you begin any type of exercise program, have a medical examination by a doctor, and have a saliva adrenal and thyroid hormone test by your Clinical Nutritionist.

1. Make an appointment with yourself. Get out your calendar right now and mark in three to four days a week that you will exercise, what you will do, and for how long.

2. Go slow. For many people the only exercise they've done recently is running through their mail! Most people think they have to push and shove their bodies in ways they just can't. You don't have to do high impact aerobics to make up for lost years.

3. Start with something you like and can do (for a lifetime). Have fun! Experiment. Many people start with walking like I did. When I felt strong enough, I progressed to jogging, then running, and, later, aerobics. Walking is easy, safe, cheap, requires no specific equipment, can be done all year round, indoors and outdoors, and, most of all, it's natural.

4. Find a partner. This is especially important if you're the kind who needs someone to go with you to keep you on track. Having a friend to workout with will help you stay motivated on the days when you don't feel like working out.

5. Adjust your attitude. Change your mind about exercise! Don't think about the inconvenience of exercise; think about the results you will be getting!

Don't focus on how out of shape you are, but keep your mind occupied by listening to inspirational or educational tapes.

I used to write out my goals on a 3 by 5 card and then meditate on them while exercising. I've learned to take a small pen and notebook with me when I walk because I get so many inspired ideas that I don't want to forget.

When your mind (and mouth) is preoccupied with uplifting thoughts that require you to imagine pictures and events, you cannot, at the same time, think about how lousy your body feels or those aches and pains from not working out!

Of course, if you feel any sharp, consistent pain, stop exercising and check with your physician or personal trainer before proceeding. Okay, let's wrap up this book with a chapter on how to put it all together.

Chapter Eleven

How Can I Get Started?

You've read about energy and all of the factors that can make us tired. You understand the link between nutrition and fatigue. But now, you may feel exhausted! Where do you begin?

My first goal with every client is to keep their blood sugar level normal. So in this chapter, I'll give you an eating plan that will help you.

1. Plan your weekly meals.

At the end of this chapter, I'll give you High Energy Meal Planning followed by Sample Meals and a short Glycemic Index Chart (see pages 82 and 104). Most people feel overwhelmed when they first start planning meals. Here are some additional planning tips:

a. Find a time to plan your meals for the week, for example, an hour on a Saturday or Sunday afternoon.

b. Write out the meals you want to make for the week on a calendar or notebook.

c. Make a shopping list of the foods needed for these recipes. Inventory the foods you have on hand, and go over each recipe, jotting down the type and amount of foods you need.

d. Take the list with you and buy the foods you need for the week.

2. Plan your 15 minute "quiet time" for stress management. Consciously plan the first 10 or 15 minutes of your day to set a positive attitude.

3. Plan your exercise time. If you don't plan it, you won't do it! Get out a calendar and mark the four or five times you can follow your 30-40 minute exercise program.

4. Take the recommended supplements.

Review the nutritional tests (pages 18, 30, 37 and 48) and note the one where you scored the highest. This is the area where you will want to focus.

Chapter One: Chronic Fatigue/Fibromyalgia

Recommended supplements:

·Antioxidants (vitamins A, C, E and selenium)
·Magnesium
·Vitamin B complex
·Folic acid/B12 and Iron (per test results)
·Essential oils (Omega 3 fats)
·Zinc and chromium
·Gymnema (Medi-Herb)

Chapter Two: Adrenal Stress

Recommended supplements:

·Vitamin B complex
·Magnesium
·Essential oils
·Eleuthero Root (Siberian Ginseng) (Medi-Herb)
·Panax Ginseng (Medi-Herb)
·Licorice Root (Medi-Herb)
·Withania (Ashwaganda by Medi-Herb)
·Antioxidants (vitamins A, C, E and selenium)
· Desiccated adrenal support

Chapter Three: Depression and Low Thyroid

Recommended supplements for low thyroid:

·Iodine or kelp

·Selenium and Magnesium

·Vitamin B complex

·Essential oils (Omega 3 fats)

·Desiccated Thyroid Supplement

·Antioxidants

Recommended supplements for depression:

·Vitamin B complex and Folic acid/B12

·Essential oils (Omega 3 fats)

·Ginkgo

·St. John's Wort

·Probiotics and liver detox

Chapter Four: Low Blood Sugar

Recommended supplements:

·Chromium GTF and Zinc

·Vitamin B complex

·Essential oils

·Magnesium (chocolate cravings)

·Antioxidants (vitamins A, C, E and selenium)

·Gymnema

Chapter Five: Insomnia

Recommended supplements:

·Calcium and/or magnesium

·Zinc, chromium and gymnema

·Vitamin B and C complex

·Essential oils (Omega 3 fats)

·Valerian Root or St. John's Wort

·Liver detoxification program

Chapter Six: Digestion

Recommended supplements:

·Digestive enzymes

·Probiotics

·Vitamin B complex

·Essential oils

·Fiber

High Energy Meal Planning Tips

·Eat every 2-3 hours which helps maintain normal blood-sugar levels. Try not to skip meals.

·Drink one half your body weight in ounces of pure water.

·Balance protein with complex carbohydrates and essential fats.

·Eat real, whole foods such as fruits and vegetables at least two meals daily (5-7 servings).

·Try to eat protein and carbohydrates with each meal; don't eat carbohydrates alone.

·Take one tablespoon of flaxseed oil daily or three portions of salmon weekly.

·Avoid processed, artificial, fake, fried and junk foods.

·Avoid soda, caffeine and desserts and other stimulants.

·Try to eat 5-6 mini-meals daily, or small meals plus snacks.

·Use sea salt. Your adrenal glands need salt for health and a small amount won't cause high blood pressure.

Sample Meals

Breakfast

1. Oatmeal or Oat Bran (with small amount of protein like egg or cottage cheese) OR
2. Protein Drink or Protein Drink Smoothie OR
3. Eggs with one slice of whole grain toast and butter

Lunch

Try to have a large vegetable dish, animal or vegetable protein and one-half to one serving of a complex carbohydrate.

Choose from:

1. Vegetable salad, grilled chicken strips (or vegetarian protein) and one slice of whole grain bread

2. Stir-fried vegetables, baked salmon and one-half cup of brown rice

3. Steamed vegetables, turkey breast (or tempeh or tofu), and one slice of whole grain bread or a baked yam

Dressing: Make an olive oil, lemon dressing. (See *Why Can't I Lose Weight Cookbook?* for great recipes.)

Dinner

Same as lunch. Try to have a large vegetable dish, animal or vegetable protein and one-half to one serving of a complex carbohydrate.

Snacks

1 boiled egg

1 nectarine with cottage cheese

1 apple with a handful of raw almonds

Eliminate These Foods and Beverages

- White sugar and snack foods made with white sugar
- White flour and foods made with white flour
- Fast food and fried foods
- Processed and refined foods
- Hydrogenated and partially hydrogenated fats (such as margarine and Crisco)
- Processed vegetable oils
- Preserved meats such as: bacon, salami, hot dogs and sausage
- Caffeine, alcohol, soft drinks, diet colas & carbonated drinks
- Chocolate and chocolate-based products, dyed teas
- French fries, corn products, potatoes, and potato chips

For energy and weight loss, choose foods with a low Glycemic Index. (see page 80.)

Sample Glycemic Index Chart

Vegetables

Low: Tomatoes, green peas, artichoke, broccoli, asparagus, brussels sprouts, cauliflower, cucumber

Medium: Yams, frozen peas, beets

High: Instant and microwaved potatoes

Grains

Low: Oat bran and slow cooking cereals, Pumpernickel

Medium: Grape Nuts, Cream of Wheat, Brown rice

High: Instant, flaked and puffed cereals, white breads

Fruits

Low: Cherries, peaches, plums, pears, apples

Medium: Juices, oranges, sweetened prunes

High: Sugar sweetened fruit juice, ripe bananas, dried raisins, mango and pineapple

Beans

Low: Lentils, chick peas, navy beans, black-eyed peas

Medium: Pinto, kidney beans, baked beans

High: Canned beans with sugar

Snacks

Low: Peanuts, almonds, walnuts

Medium: Microwave popcorn, wheat crackers

High: Potato chips, rice cakes, sugar-sweetened snacks

A Final Word

Be encouraged that making the suggested changes can and will help you gain your health and energy back. No matter what steps you begin to take, realize that they all will help, and it's worth the effort!

May God bless you on your journey to health and energy!

Endnotes

1. Jacob Teitelbaum, M.D. *From Fatigued to Fantastic* (New York, NY: Penguin Putnam, 2001), p. 2.

2. Centers for Disease Control and Prevention: December 1994.

3. Ronald L. Hoffman, M.D., *Tired All the Time: How To Regain Your Lost Energy* (New York: NY: Pocket Books, 1993), p. 215.

4. Teitelbaum, p. 5.

5. Lorna R. Vanderhaeghe and Patrick J.D. Bouic, Ph.D., *The Immune System Cure* (New York, NY: Kensington Books, 1999), p. 193.

6. Teitelbaum, p. 2.

7. Harris H. McIlwain, M.D., and Debra Fulghum Bruce, *The Fibromyalgia Handbook* (New York, NY: Henry Holt and Co., Inc., 1996), p. 16.

8. E. Eolfe, et. al., "The American College of Rheumatology 1990 Criteria for the Classification of Fibromyalgia: Report of the Multicenter Criteria Committee," *Arthritis and Rheumatology* 33 (1990):160-172.

9. Dr. Joe Elrod, *Reversing Fibromyalgia* (Pleasant Grove, Utah: Woodland Publishing, 2002) p. 27.

10. Dr. Bruce West, *Health Alert,* Vol. 15, Issue 4, p. 1.

11. Dr. Bruce West, *Health Alert,* Vol. 15, Issue 4, p. 2.

12. Stephen Astor, M.D., *Hidden Food Allergies* (Garden City, NY: Avery Publishing, 1988, 1997), p. 1.

13. Dr. Joseph Mercola, web address www.mercola.com.

14. Elrod, p. 16.

15. Holmes, T. & Rabe, R. (1967) "Holmes-Rabe Social Readjustment Rating Scale," *Journal of Psychosomatic Research,* Vol. II.

16. Diana Schwarzbein, M.D., *The Schwarzbein Principle II* (Deerfield Beach, FL: Health Communications, Inc., 2002), p. 127.

17. Dr. James Wilson, *Adrenal Fatigue: The 21st Century Stress Syndrome* (Petaluma, CA: Smart Publications, 2001) pp. 8-9.

18. Maureen Salaman, *Your Health Questions Answered Naturally* (Mountain View, CA: MKS, Inc., 1998), p. 612, 988.

19. Schwarzbein, pp. 361-379.

20. Wilson, p. 51.

21. Wilson, p. 53.

22. Ibid.

23. Leon Chaitow, N.D., D.O., *You Don't Have to Die: Unraveling the AIDS Myth* (Puyallup, Washington: Future Medicine Publishing, Inc., 1994), p. 74-75.

24. Salaman, p. 114.

25. Wilson, p. 236.

26. Lorrie Medford, *Why Can't I Lose Weight?* (Tulsa, OK: LDN Publishing, 1999), p. 69.

27. Broda O. Barnes, M.D. *Hypothyroidism: The Unsuspected Illness* (New York, NY: Harper and Row, 1976), pp. 42-48.

28. The Eck Newsletter, January, 1999.

29. Carol Simontacchi, C.N., *Crazy Makers: How the Food Industry is Destroying Our Brains and Harming Our Children* (New York, NY: Penguin Putnam, Inc., 2000), p. 25.

30. Dr. John Lee, *Medical Letter,* July 2001.

31. American Psychiatric Association, Web address www.psych.org.

32. Martin Budd, N.D., D.O., *Why Am I So Tired: Is Your Thyroid Making You Ill?* (Hammersmith, London: Harper Collins, 2000), pp. 46-47.

33. Dr. John Lee, July 2001, p. 2.

34. Schwarzbein, pp. 64, 70, 132-136.

35. Dr. Bruce West, *Health Alert,* Vol. 19, Issue 1, p. 6.

36. Marcia Zimmerman, C.N. *The A.D.D. Nutrition Solution: A Drug-Free 30-Day Plan* (New York, NY: Henry Holt and Co., 1999), p. 85.

37. Wilson, p. 237.

38. John Lee, M.D., *Medical Letter,* July 2001, p. 2.

39. Ibid.

40. John Lee, M.D., *Medical Letter,* Dec. 2002, p. 2.

41. John Lee, M.D. *Medical Letter,* May 2001, p. 3.

42. Nancy Appleton, Ph.D., *Lick the Sugar Habit* (Garden City Park, NY: Avery Publishing Group, 1988), p. 21 (Web address: www.nancyappleton.com).

43. Mary Jane Parks, *A New You* (Frankfort, KY: Parks Publishers, 1982), p. 24.

44. Ann Louise Gittleman, *Get the Sugar Out* (New York, NY: Crown Trade Paperbacks), 1996, p. xiii.

45. Dr. Bruce West, *Health Alert,* Vol. 16, Issue 2, p. 1.

46. Ibid.

47. Earl Mindell, Ph.D., *Prescription Alternatives* (Los Angeles, CA: Keats Publishing, 1998), p. 401.

48. Dr. Bruce West, *Health Alert Report,* "Secret Link Between Indigestion and Disease," p. 38.

49. Dr. Bruce West, *Disease and Prevention,* (Monterey, CA, 1995), p. 14.

50. Mindell, p. 367.

51. *Journal of Clinical Endocrinology and Metabolism,* August 2001; 86:3787-3794.

52. Annual Meeting of American Diabetes Assn., June 25, 2001, Philadelphia.

53. *Journal of the American Medical Association,* Nov. 1, 2000; p. 284.

54. *Lancet,* October 23, 1999; 354:1435-1439.

55. Dr. Jonn Matsen, *The Mysterious Cause of Illness* (Canfield, OH: Fischer Publishing, 1987), pp. 7-9.

56. William G. Crook, *Chronic Fatigue Syndrome and the Yeast Connection* (New York, NY: Vintage Books, 1986), p. 133.

57. Dr. Don Colbert, *What You Don't Know May Be Killing You* (Lake Mary, FL: Siloam Press, 2000), p. 151.

58. Luc De Schepper, M.D., Ph.D., C.A., *Peak Immunity: How To Fight Epstein-Barr Virus, Candida, Herpes Simplex and other Immuno-Depressive Disorders and Win* (Santa Monica, CA, 1989), p. 80.

59. Mindell, p. 285.

60. Dr. John Lee, *Medical Letter,* Nov. 2001, p. 2.

61. *Science Magazine,* August 92, 257:1036-1038.

62. Dr. Michael Schmidt, *Beyond Antibiotics* (Berkeley, CA: North Atlantic Books, 1993), p. 26.

63. Dr. John Lee, *Medical Letter*, Sept/Oct. 2001, p. 4.

64. Dr. Bruce West, *Health Alert*, Volume 16, Issue 9.

65. Simontacchi, p. 15.

66. Sally Fallon, *Nourishing Traditions:The Cookbook that Challenges Politically Correct Nutrition and the Diet Dictocrats* (Washington, D.C.: New Trends Publishing, Inc.,1999, 2001) p. 3.

67. Dr. Robert Arnot, *The Breast Cancer Prevention Diet* (New York, NY: Little, Brown and Co., 1998), p. xiii.

68. Marion Burros, "Additives in Advice on Food?" *New York Times,* Nov. 15, 1995, Vol. 145, p. C1.

69. Sally Fallon, "Diet and Heart Disease: Not What You Think," *Consumers' Research,* July 1996, p. 19.

70. Dr. Royal Lee, "How and Why Synthetic Poisons Are Being Sold as Imitations of Natural Foods and Drugs," December 1948.

71. Schwarzbein, M.D., *The Schwarzbein Principle* (Deerfield Beach, FL: Health Communications, Inc., 1999), p. 71.

72. Ibid.

73. Medford, p. 90.

74. Dr. Royal Lee, "The Special Nutritional Qualities of Natural Foods": 1942, Report No. 4, pp. 38-39.

75. Paul Addis, *Food and Nutrition News,* March/April 1990, 62:2:7-10.

76. Schwarzbein, p. 61.

77. Schwarzbein, p. 71.

78. Dr. Royal Lee, pp. 38-39.

79. Ibid.

80. Ibid.

81. Medford, p. 245.

82. Medford, p. 170.

I have made every effort possible to check the accuracy of material quoted. If there is any question, or a possible mistake in quoting of any material, necessary changes will be made in future editions.

Index

A

Aches, 20, 30, 98
Acidophilus, 65
ADD (Attention Deficit Disorder), 44
Addiction, 73
Addison's disease, 30, 31
Adrenal, fatigue, 15, 19, 25-36, 37, 59
Adrenal glands, 15, 25-36, 37, 49, 73
Adrenal hormones, 32, 35, 59
Adult onset diabetes, 31, 53
Aerobic exercise, 97
Alarm response, 28
Alcohol, 28, 31, 34, 46, 48, 55, 70, 73, 87, 90, 103
Allergies, 13, 19-23, 51, 58, 71
Ambien, 58
American Dietetic Association (ADA), 69
Anemia, 13, 19, 84-86
Antacids, 61
Antibiotics, 16, 62-65
Anti-depressants, 14, 20, 22, 31, 32, 40, 41, 43, 45, 72
Antioxidants, 35, 40, 46, 55, 74, 79, 87, 101
Anxiety, 18, 20, 21, 29-31, 33, 34, 44, 45, 50, 58, 81, 86, 96, 100
Armour, thyroid, 43
Artificial sweeteners, 53
Aspartame, 31, 34, 70
Arthritis, 38, 51

B

B complex vitamins, 33, 34, 44, 45, 55, 84, 85, 91, 100-102
Bacteria, friendly, good (see acidophilus), 62-65
Barnes, Dr. Broda, 38-39
Barnes Basal Temperature Test, 39
Bioflavonoids, 46
Birth control pills, 86
Blood pressure, 29, 30, 37, 40, 48, 49, 51, 58, 60, 70, 95
Blood sugar, 13, 14, 30, 46-49, 55, 70, 80, 88, 89, 91, 95
Bowel, irritable, 20
Brain fog, 11, 18, 25, 37, 41

C

Caffeine (coffee), 14, 27, 28, 31, 33, 34, 37, 41, 44, 46, 59, 60, 70, 73, 81, 85, 87, 90, 101-103
Calcium, 50, 60, 85, 88, 90
Cancer, 49, 50, 54, 68, 69, 74, 83, 84, 96
Carbohydrates, 13, 34, 48, 49, 54, 55, 59, 70-73, 75, 76, 79-81, 89, 97, 101, 102
Carrots, 46
Centers for Disease Control (CDC), 18, 64
Cholesterol, 19, 37, 38, 40, 49, 50, 51, 54, 69, 70, 74, 75, 86, 96, 101
Chromium, 35, 50, 54, 55, 88, 102
Chronic Fatigue Syndrome (CFS), 13, 18, 19, 25, 31, 42, 57, 61, 63, 100
Chronic infections, (See infections)
Citrus, 22, 28
Coffee, 28, 29, 34, 39, 48, 73, 77, 81, 91
Colon cancer, 50
Cortisol, 29, 30, 32, 73, 90
Constipation, 13, 23, 37, 38, 52, 62, 65
Cushing's disease, 31

D

Deficiencies, 13, 14, 17, 19, 20, 21, 23, 29, 42, 44, 59, 70, 81, 83-85, 87
Depression, 12, 14, 15, 18, 20, 21, 23, 25, 26, 29-31, 37-40, 42-44, 46, 48, 52, 58, 60, 70, 81, 86, 95, 100, 101
Detoxification, 40, 60
DHEA, 32, 35
Diabetes, 13, 19, 29, 31, 38, 48, 53, 54, 55, 60, 68, 83, 96, 102
Diet, poor, 13, 19, 21, 23, 34, 49, 59, 92
Diet, vegetarian, 73
Dietary Goals of the U.S., 25
Digestive enzymes, 65, 77
Digestive problems, 23, 30, 61, 68, 71
Disease, 13, 15, 21, 23, 25, 28, 29, 31, 32, 33, 38, 40, 46, 48, 50, 52, 53, 55, 59, 61-62, 64, 68-75, 79, 83, 84, 88, 95, 96
Drugs, 13, 22, 31-33, 40, 41, 43-46, 54, 57, 59, 64, 65-70

E

Effexor, 40
Eggs, 44, 74, 86, 89, 102, 103
Energy, 11, 15, 17, 23, 25, 28, 29, 33, 34, 42, 55, 57, 58, 61, 65, 67, 70, 71, 73, 76-80, 82, 84, 86-89, 94-96, 99, 101, 104
Enzymes, 52, 61, 77, 102
Epstein Barr virus (EBV), 13, 18
Essential fatty acids (EFAs), 22, 54, 55, 80, 102
Estrogen, 36, 39, 41, 82
Exercise, 12, 15, 17, 18, 23, 27, 31, 33, 37, 43, 46, 49, 53, 54, 55, 70, 82, 89, 90, 91, 93-96, 98, 99

F

Fat-free, 28
Fatigue, 11, 12-15, 17-23, 25, 27, 29, 37, 38, 41, 42, 47-50, 56-63, 65, 68, 70, 72, 73, 77, 79, 82-84, 86-88, 91, 95, 96, 99, 100
Fats and Fatty acids (See essential fatty acids)
Ferritin, 85
Fertility, 38
Fiber, 62, 81, 102
Fibromyalgia, 15, 20-23, 31, 57, 61
Fight or flight response, 28
Fish oil, 102
Flaxseeds, oil, 22, 46, 55, 80, 102
Folate (folic acid), 34, 40, 85-87, 100
Food Allergies, 19, 21, 22, 51
Food and Drug Administration (FDA), 43, 53
Food Pyramid, 72
Free Radicals, 35, 51, 74, 85

G

Garlic, 40
Ginkgo, 46, 101
Ginseng, 35, 46, 100
Glucose Tolerance Factor, 88
Glycemic Index, 55, 79, 80, 99, 104
Grains, whole, 34, 35, 80, 89, 103
Grave's disease, 42

H

HDL (high-density lipoproteins), 50, 96
Hair loss, 29, 37
Headaches, 18, 20, 22, 29, 30, 48, 52, 58
Heartburn, 22, 30
Heart disease, 13, 19, 29, 48, 50, 51, 68-70, 72, 74, 83, 84-86, 88, 96, 97
Hemorrhoids, 51
High-blood pressure, 20, 40, 48, 58, 60, 70
High cholesterol, 37, 40, 54, 70, 74, 75, 86
Homocysteine, 86
Hormones, 28, 29, 32, 35, 41, 42, 60, 70, 74, 89
Hydrochloric acid, 61, 65, 85, 86
Hypertension, 29, 38, 52, 88
Hypoglycemia, 13, 19, 30, 31, 38, 48, 50, 55, 89
Hypothyroidism, 19, 37-39, 42, 43, 45, 82, 85

I

Immune system, 19, 21, 63-65, 84, 96
Infections, 18, 19, 21, 31, 38, 58, 64, 100
Insomnia, 13, 14, 29-31, 35, 37, 42, 45, 57-60, 89, 90, 101
Insulin, 15, 31, 49, 51-53, 60, 70-76, 79, 88, 89, 94, 95-97
Iodine, 39, 101
Iron, 84, 85, 100

J-K

Journal of Medicine, 41
Journal of Endocrinology, 59
Journal of the American Medical Association, 60
Journal of Clinical Nutrition, 83
Kava, 46, 91
Kelp, 101
Kidney, 28, 48, 49-52, 60, 62, 81, 104

L

LDL, (low-density lipoprotein), 49, 50
Lee, John, Dr., 41, 43, 46, 49, 64, 65
Lee, Royal, Dr., 69, 72, 75
Licorice root, 100
Liver, 13, 23, 35, 40, 46, 49, 52, 54, 57, 60, 62, 71, 76, 77, 84, 85, 86, 88, 101
Low-blood sugar, 13, 14, 30, 37, 48, 49, 89

M

Magnesium, 23, 34, 35, 50, 54, 60, 88, 90, 100, 101
Malnourished, 45
Manganese, 34
Margarine, 68, 74, 75, 80, 103
Melatonin, 89, 91, 94
Memory, 30, 44, 46, 87
Mercury, toxicity, 39

Metabolism, 12, 21, 37, 39, 54, 55, 59, 60, 88, 95

N

Naps, need for, 90
Nicotine, 28, 96
Nitrates, 34

O

Olive, oil, 75, 80, 103
Omega 3 fats, 45, 46, 75

P

Panic attacks, 29, 33, 35, 93
Pernicious anemia, 85, 86
Processed foods, 27, 39, 40, 53, 55, 62, 67-70, 83, 93
Progesterone, 41
Prozac, 40, 72, 89
Protein, 31, 35, 51, 54, 70, 72, 76, 78-81, 85, 86, 89, 102, 103

Q-R

Recommended Daily Allowance (RDA), 84
Riboflavin, 34

S

St. John's Wort, 40, 41, 45, 91, 101
Salmon, 34, 55, 75, 80, 102, 103
Saturated fat, 68, 80
Serotonin, 21, 23, 43, 45, 50, 71, 72, 76, 81, 89, 94, 95
Sleep, 18-21, 25, 27, 30, 32, 41, 42, 45, 55-60, 69, 89, 90, 91, 94
Standard Process, 55, 65, 81, 88
Stevia, 49, 71, 81
Stimulants, 14, 28, 33, 34, 37, 43-46, 60, 72, 73, 76, 90, 102
Stress, 13, 15, 21, 22, 23, 25-35, 39, 44, 45, 49, 52, 59, 60, 72, 73, 83, 87, 89, 91-93, 94, 96, 99, 100
Sugar, 21, 22, 27, 28, 29, 33, 34, 39, 41, 45, 47-55, 59, 60, 62, 68,73, 75, 76, 78-82, 87, 88, 91, 95, 99, 101-104
Supplements, 12, 15, 21, 23, 33-35, 41, 42, 43, 45, 46, 54, 55, 73, 80-88, 94, 101-104
Synthroid, 43

T

Test, nutrition, 18, 30, 37, 48
Thiamine, 34, 84
Thyroid, 13-15, 19, 33, 35, 37-39, 41-43, 45-47, 57, 59, 60, 76, 82, 85, 95, 97, 100, 101
Thyroxine, 38
Trans fats, 74, 80
Trigger points, 20

U-V

U.S.D.A. (United States Department of Agriculture), 72, 84
Valerian root, 91, 101
Virus, 13, 18, 19, 29, 62, 63, 64
Vitamins:
A, 35
B, 33, 45, 55, 84, 85, 101, 102
C, 35, 79, 84, 85
D, 75
E, 35

W

White flour, 55, 68, 69, 71, 72, 103
Whole-food supplements, 21, 42, 88, 94
Why Am I So Wacky?, 41
Why Can't I Lose Weight?, 63, 77
Why Can't I Lose Weight Cookbook, 78, 103
Why Can't I Stay Motivated?, 82
Why Do I Feel So Lousy?, 40, 60, 65, 77
Why Do I Need Whole-Food Supplements?, 21, 34, 87, 88

X-Y-Z

Yeast infections, 62, 63
Zinc, 54, 87, 100, 101

Order Form

Please Print

Name ______________________________

Address ______________________________

City ____________________ State _____ Zip __________

Phone ______________________________

E-mail ______________________________

METHOD OF PAYMENT

Check ____ Credit Card: Visa_____ Mastercard_____

Card number ____________________ Exp. date_______

Authorization Signature ____________________

ITEM	QTY	PRICE
Why Can't I Lose Weight? ($17.95)		
Why Can't I Lose Weight Cookbook ($17.95)		
Why Can't I Stay Motivated? ($14.95)		
Why Am I So Grumpy, Dopey and Sleepy? ($11.95)		
Why Am I So Wacky? ($11.95)		
Why Eat Like Jesus Ate? ($11.95)		
Why Do I Need Whole Food Supplements? ($9.95)		
Why Do I Feel So Lousy? ($9.95)		
Why Do I Really Need Herbs? ($9.95)		
Subtotal		
Shipping & Handling		
Add 15%		
(Add 8% if resident of OK) Tax		
Total		

Send check or money order to:

Life Design Nutrition
Lorrie Medford, CN
PO Box 54007
Tulsa, OK 74155
918-664-4483
918-664-0300 (fax)
E-mail orders: lorrie@lifedesignnutrition.com
www.lifedesignnutrition.com